Cash Cow

Cash Cow

Ten Myths about the Dairy Industry

ÉLISE DESAULNIERS

Translated by Marie-Claude Plourde
Revised by Elisabeth Lyman

Lantern Books ● New York
A Division of Booklight Inc.

2015
Lantern Books
128 Second Place
Brooklyn, NY 11231
www.lanternbooks.com

We thank SODEC for its support for the English translation of this book.

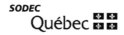

Front cover image: Dairy cow in Sweden 2012, © Jo-Anne McArthur. Used with permission.

Printed in the United States of America

Library of Congress Cataloging-in-Publication Data

Desaulniers, Élise, author.
  [Vache à lait. English]
  Cash cow : ten myths about the dairy industry / Elise Desaulniers ; translated by Marie-Claude Plourde ; revised by Elisabeth Lyman.
      pages cm
  Includes bibliographical references.
  ISBN 978-1-59056-493-6 (pbk. : alk. paper)—ISBN 978-1-59056-494-3 (ebooks)
  1. Dairy products industry—Quebec (Province) 2. Dairy products in human nutrition. 3. Milk consumption—Social aspects. I. Title.
  HD9275.C3Q417513 2015
  338.4'763709714--dc23

                                      2015030943

To Jersey cow no. 67

"There is probably more suffering in a glass of milk or an ice cream cone than there is in a steak."
—**Gary L. Francione**, philosopher and legal scholar, 2008

"Our strategy is twofold: a rational approach and an emotional approach. The former presents milk as a significant source of calcium and a first-choice weapon in the fight against osteoporosis, while the latter showcases the joyful reunion of consumers and milk."
—**Nicole Dubé**, marketing director, Quebec Federation of Milk Producers, 2002

"Cow's milk has become a point of controversy among doctors and nutritionists. There was a time when it was considered very desirable [to drink milk], but research has forced us to rethink this recommendation. . . . Dairy products contribute to a surprising number of health problems."
—**Benjamin Spock, M.D.**, pediatrician and author, 1998

"Élise! Drink your glass of milk before you leave the table."
—**Édith Desaulniers**, mother, 1979

Contents

Élise Desaulniers and the Democratic Conversation

W HAT KIND OF READER WILL learn the most from this fine book? The one who knows nothing about the subject it covers, or the one who knows it all too well? Between the two, I admit it's hard to decide.

Most certainly, the first type will learn many things—often astonishing and unfortunately very sad—about the dairy industry, the animals that are its main victims, and what is kept hidden from us, not to mention its strategies aimed at winning us over and manipulating us. Élise Desaulniers is an excellent teacher, providing clear explanations and arguments backed by solid references. This book's strongest point is that it helps us understand so many things. And that's extremely important.

But people who already know everything (or almost everything) about the topic will still learn some very important things from this book, especially in terms of how such controversial topics should be addressed—topics that some may find disturbing and contentious—and how to include them in the democratic conversation. As I see it, we can learn an enormous amount from the author in this respect. We can all, myself included, benefit a great deal from reflecting upon this issue, especially given today's political climate.

This distressing phenomenon is well known and I will not dwell on it here. Let us just remember that there is good reason to believe that between the propagandistic goals of the dominant institutions and the active omnipresence of public relations firms, our democratic conversation is now facing real and dramatic challenges. But these already significant difficulties are increased tenfold when it comes to including topics that many find controversial or disturbing and trying to initiate dialogue about them. This is particularly true if the dominant institutions find these issues inconvenient: global warming and the ethics of our economic institutions are two examples.

Those who attempt to publicly discuss such topics and raise such questions are likely to fail. Overcoming our society's resistance requires a lot of finesse, delicacy, and intelligence.

In my opinion, Élise Desaulniers is a model to emulate in this regard. She manages to inform without confronting, to teach without indoctrinating. She invites us to reflect on issues that can have a significant impact on our lives, but she does this with modesty, without lecturing, and in an inviting way that allows her admirable humanity and sensitivity to shine through.

In these pages, you will see, for example, how elegantly she presents herself, admitting that there have been occasions on which she also succumbed to the illusions she hopes to free us from. You will be encouraged by the way she continually mentions her own hesitations and doubts: all of this is what makes you actually want to listen to what she has to say.

These strengths of hers made a big impression on me when I read her first book. I was delighted to find my positive feeling about her unchanged after reading this second one.

But I am also delighted by this author's work because I suspect that on the issue of animal ethics we have probably reached—or are about to reach—what I like to call a moral tipping point.

It is clear that our ethical standards evolve with time, and that we gradually include new questions, problems, and even beings in the sphere of ethics. This is how a few formerly common practices, like corporal punishment at schools, have now become unacceptable for ethical reasons. We could easily cite many other examples in which similar changes to accepted practices have occurred.

There comes a time when the untenable nature of certain practices, recognized initially by only a few reformers, starts to become obvious to more and more people. Then comes the moment—and this is the famous tipping point—when the majority of society agrees with what only bold precursors originally supported. When it comes to animal ethics, I think we're getting there.

I strongly suspect that, a few decades from now, our descendants will wonder how we could have treated animals the way we do today. If so, inquiring into these issues and deciding for ourselves how we should respond to the situation is a moral duty that each of us ought to take very seriously.

It would be difficult to find a better guide and traveling companion for this task than Élise Desaulniers.

—**Normand Baillargeon**, *Professor, Université du Québec à Montréal*

Foreword

Beyond the Pail

ÉLISE DESAULNIERS' *CASH COW* OFFERS lots of valuable insights into the role that the dairy industry plays in the agricultural economies of North America and how deeply intertwined are the consumption and promotion of dairy products with concepts of appropriate nutrition, early childhood education, and regional and even national identity. She also effectively calls out the arguments for dairy consumption for what they are: often false and almost wholly determined by industry demands for profits and dominance, not good science or public policy.

The social, political, psychological, and economic complexities of our relationship with food, the environment, and other animals have long been a concern of mine and the non-profit policy "action" tank I founded, Brighter Green, headquartered in New York.

For several years, Brighter Green has been examining the effects of intensive animal agriculture on food security, public health, natural resources, deforestation and biodiversity loss, animal and human welfare, and climate change from a global perspective. Brighter Green has studied how large-scale cultivation of soybeans for animal feed and industrial production of beef, chicken, and pork are negatively affecting the rainforest and the tropical savanna of Brazil; the environmental, public health, and ethical problems posed by China's intensification of its pork industry; India's expansion and industrialization of poultry and dairy production; and the growth of factory farm–style facilities in Ethiopia, despite myriad and persistent ecological and food security challenges.

We've detailed alternatives to the current trajectories of seemingly inevitable growth and industrialization, and are liaising with an increasing number of organizations and individuals around the world who are challenging the power of the livestock and feed sectors. Brighter Green also recently published an in-depth examination of the emergence of industrialized dairy systems across Asia and its consequences for the environment, public health, livelihoods, and the cows themselves. I believe the findings will be of interest to readers of *Cash Cow* since the process and results (so far) of selling the "dairy dream" in Asia reflect what Élise documents from her North American experience. I draw from this research for the text that follows.

Cash Cow illustrates well how passionately many Quebecers and Canadians love their dairy products! The fact is, however, that because markets for dairy products in developed countries such as Canada and the United States have reached a virtual saturation point, the dairy industry is seeking to expand into other markets, most notably in Asia. At first glance, as Élise's research suggests, this may seem counter-intuitive. Traditional diets in East Asian countries include virtually no or a negligible amount of dairy. When dairy is eaten, it's almost always only by infants or young children. Not surprisingly, lactose intolerance is widespread across East Asia.

Nonetheless, neither the lack of a cultural or dietary tradition of consuming milk and dairy, nor the risks to individual well-being of eating dairy despite having difficulty digesting lactose, have stopped the drive of "cash cows" across the region. This is a result of both supply and demand, and, in line with Élise's findings, in no small measure, skillful marketing. Due to their fast-growing populations and rising incomes, China, India, and several countries in Southeast Asia are receiving attention and investment from international and domestic dairy producers that are either operating, or aiming to operate, at an industrial scale.

An "untapped" emerging market of nearly three billion potential new dairy consumers exists across the global South. This conclusion was reached through research by Tetra Pak, which pioneered the use of aseptic packaging. Tetra Pak–insulated paper cartons will be familiar to anyone who drinks soy, almond, or other non-dairy milks. (The packaging means it's not necessary to refrigerate the container to keep the liquid inside from spoiling.) But Tetra Pak is also the world's leading producer of packaging for pasteurized dairy products—and refrigeration for foodstuffs in retail shops and homes, especially in rural areas, is still relatively rare in many parts of Asia.

To dairy promoters, Asia represents a vast pool of potential new consumers.[1] China and India together are home to more than 2.5 billion people. The rapid expansion of U.S.

fast food chains across Asia is also raising demand for dairy products and the "reliable" supply chains industrialized dairy operations purport to provide. At the same time, school milk programs, many sponsored by multinational food companies with dairy divisions, such as Nestlé, have become popular in a number of countries. Government support (as in the U.S. and Canada) makes these program not only viable, but also often unavoidable.

Amid the rush to reach unexploited markets, and in the rise of consumer culture, public health concerns have largely been set aside. It's a rather sinister consequence of lactose intolerance combined with more people drinking milk or eating processed dairy foods, that another new market has been created: over-the-counter aids to help individuals digest dairy.

By 2025, countries in the global South are expected to devour nearly twice as much milk and milk products as they did in 1997, rising to 375 million metric tons from 194 million metric tons.[2] Asia is already the world's highest dairy-consuming region, with 39 percent of global consumption, due mainly to China and India, the world's two most populous countries, as well as Pakistan, which has a large population and, akin to India, high levels of milk consumption.[3] Rates of dairy consumption across Asia vary widely, from 11.5 kilograms (kg) (25 pounds/lb) of milk per person a year in Viet Nam to 30 kg (66 lb) a year in China and 72 kg (159 lb) per capita each year in India (2009 data).[4] As of now, these levels remain below those in industrialized nations.[5] If the industry has anything to do with it, however, this will change, and rapidly.

For instance, in China, domestic production of milk is expected to triple by 2030—part of a policy of expansion that has been underway since the 1990s. I have Chinese colleagues in their twenties who tell me that when they were in school all they were given to drink was (cows') "milk, milk, milk," and that they rarely even saw water. The Chinese government and large numbers of Chinese individuals have come to believe that dairy is important for good health and to ensuring that kids grow up to be big and strong (mirroring Élise's exploration of the roots of high dairy consumption in Canada and other industrialized countries).

Cambodia now has several KFCs, as well as burger and pizza chains; all feature meat and dairy in abundance. KFC's menu in Cambodia includes "cheezy wedges" alongside fried chicken. A Cambodian medical doctor I know agonizes over the fast-rising incidences of diabetes in adults and even children she sees, and her patients' adoption of increasingly Westernized eating patterns: more meat, dairy products, processed and fried foods, and sugar. Until 2011, all milk and dairy products consumed in Cambodia were imported. But that year Cambodia milked its first (cash) cow, as part of a U.S. $250 million large-scale dairy facility in the southwest of the country. This industrial dairy is the result of a partnership between a Swedish dairy corporation and a Cambodian conglomerate, with support from the Cambodian government. The site borders a national park. Some environmentalists fear the park could suffer water contamination from the cows' manure. They are also concerned about possible conflicts between the dairy and the leopards and tigers who live within the park boundaries, and possible future demands for lethal "control" measures to protect the owners' investment: thousands of cows.

Well-established multinational and new regional and national dairy corporations across Asia are targeting previously unreached populations, including the rural and urban poor and school kids. Nestlé and Tetra Pak have become major players in school milk programs and classroom nutrition courses.[6] These dairy industry–influenced education initiatives facilitate the development and use of curricula biased toward dairy interests that communicate the message that consuming dairy is required for good nutrition from childhood on (a position contested by a number of public health researchers, and extensively examined by Élise in this book). Of course, school milk programs and nutritional education courses can engender lifelong habits of milk or processed dairy product consumption, strategically helping create a long-term market of industrial dairy product users—a fact that the industry is counting on.[7]

Moreover, marketing campaigns for fast food and processed dairy foods like ice cream and flavored yogurt (widely eaten by most North American children and teens) often explicitly target kids. McDonald's in India, for example, has glossy ads for its "happy meals" linking a burger and a Coke with a toy; in one ad, these toys are a dancing Barbie doll dressed in pink (presumably for Indian girls), and a red and yellow plastic hot rod car, presumably designed for boys like the one pictured with his mother, both smiling broadly.

As in the U.S., Europe, and Australia and New Zealand, "Big Dairy" in Asia has many helping hands. Unfortunately, many government policy-makers here and in other parts of the global South see the industrialized CAFO (Concentrated Animal Feeding Operations) system as necessary to meet escalating demand amid intensifying pressures on natural resources like water, land, and forests. CAFOs ("factory farms" and feedlots) are characterized by the lifelong, indoor confinement of hundreds or even thousands of animals in a single location. Although promoted as an efficient means of producing large quantities of animal products in a short time period, CAFOs have severe environmental and other consequences, as Élise shows. CAFOs create high levels of waste and pollution, affecting the livelihoods of workers and surrounding communities, contaminating soil and water supplies, and producing greenhouse gas emissions that contribute to global climate change. CAFOs also subject animals to confined spaces and numerous inhumane practices. They also give rise to zoonotic diseases, which negatively affect public health.

As Élise ably demonstrates, dairy CAFOs are no more virtuous or sustainable in this regard than factory farms for meat or egg production. Large-scale milk producers often put local dairies out of business, affecting the livelihoods of communities in rural areas. In the U.S., consolidation in the dairy sector continues, despite growing public concern. Research at U.S.-based Food & Water Watch concluded that in the fifteen years between 1997 and 2012, more than 50,000 dairies closed in the U.S. During the same fifteen years, the number of dairy operations with 500 or more cows (factory dairies) in the U.S. rose substantially, to 5.5 million from 2.5 million.[8]

A dairy CAFO with 2,500 cows creates as much waste as a city of 400,000 people, much of which is often untreated and leaches into local water supplies and ecosystems, degrading marine environments and contaminating potable water. Cows used for dairy production in CAFO systems are also resource-intensive (through no fault of their own), requiring about 15 more liters of water and significantly more feed grain than grazing cows. It takes an average of 31 liters of water to produce one gram of milk in an industrial facility. That's 50 percent more water than is required per gram for pulse (legume) protein—the traditional source of dietary protein in many Asian countries. Manure, and cows' digestive processes, are also a significant source of climate warming greenhouse gases (GHGs). The world's dairy cattle account for emissions of 1.4 gigatonnes of carbon dioxide equivalent a year—or 20 percent of the livestock sector's total GHGs.

Industrialized dairies also rely on product packaging, often single-serve varieties. Although Tetra Pak cartons are recyclable, they require specialized recycling technology that is largely unavailable in most developing countries. Dairy (and all) CAFOs create a stressful environment for the animals, which leads to high rates of hoof lesions, lameness, infections, and stomach ulcers among cows used in dairy production. Non-indigenous cows, like the Holstein-Friesian breed, are imported to Asia from New Zealand, Australia, and Uruguay because of their high milk yields, but are not adapted to the high-temperature climates and so face heat-induced stress. As Élise also observes, slaughter awaits all dairy cows—male calves usually at a very young age and their mothers and sisters once their productivity decreases.

Unlike the countries of East and Southeast Asia, India has a long tradition of milk and dairy consumption. With a vast herd of cows and buffalo, the country accounts for 16 percent of global milk production, making it the largest milk producer in the world, followed by the United States, China, Pakistan, and Brazil.[9] An irony exists in that, among Indian Hindus, the cow is sacred; and yet the pressure to produce more milk is leading to the development of dairy CAFOs in India, which will only cause further suffering to India's cattle—and not just in the extraction of milk. India today is among the global leaders in leather production (from both cows and buffalo), and, as of 2012, it had become the world's top beef exporter (largely from the meat of buffalo whose milk production has fallen from peak levels).[10] The establishment of dairy CAFOs in India means that export of cows' meat is also likely in the future.

A second irony is that the growth of industrial dairy production in Asia and other parts of the world is taking place even as a widening reevaluation is underway in industrialized countries of the desirability and sustainability of a CAFO-centered agricultural sector. Also underway is a corresponding reexamination of the health consequences of high dairy (and meat) consumption and of the need for dairy in a healthful diet, something that Élise notes extensively in *Cash Cow*.

A recent study of the U.S. dairy industry by scientists with expertise in climate change, economics, agronomy, animal welfare, and other relevant fields concluded that despite the efficiencies achieved in milk production, "the current structure of the industry lacks the resilience to adapt to changing social and environmental landscapes." One of the main challenges the researchers noted was the widening chasm between dairy industry practices and public perceptions, and a resulting decline in public trust.[11] *Cash Cow* gives considerable insight into why this has happened.

A multi-year, multi-sectoral commission on CAFOs in the U.S. assembled by the Pew Trusts concluded that this system has created "problems that are beginning to require attention by policymakers and the industry. Given the relatively rapid emergence of the technologies for industrial farm animal production, and the dependence on chemical inputs, energy, and water, many industrial farm animal production systems are not sustainable environmentally or economically."[12] In a preface to its final report, the Commission's executive director wrote that industrial farm animal production in the U.S. "presents an unacceptable level of risk to public health and damage to the environment, as well as unnecessary harm to the animals we raise for food."[13]

The growing opposition to CAFOs in industrialized countries, combined with the lack of, or lack of enforcement of, animal welfare and environmental regulations, is surely another facet of corporate dairies' interest in expanding across Asia.[14] But Big Dairy's onward global march is not a foregone conclusion. In India, China, and Southeast Asia, policymakers, civil society, and private sector investors have a chance to interrupt this cycle and create more sustainable, equitable, and humane food and agriculture systems—not least because dairy products have until recently had little dietary presence in much of East and Southeast Asia.

I hope *Cash Cow* garners a wide readership, in North America and around the world. It's a much-needed corrective to the prevailing notions of milk being both indispensable and unavoidable—*Truman Show*–like illusions that so many billions of us have been asked to swallow.

Mia MacDonald is the executive director and founder of Brighter Green, a public policy "action" tank based in Brooklyn, New York. Brighter Green works to raise awareness of and encourage policy action on issues that span the environment, animals, and sustainability. Brighter Green works in the U.S. and internationally with a focus on the countries of the global South and a strong commitment to ensuring and expanding equity and rights. This preface draws from *Beyond the Pail: The Emergence of Industrialized Dairy Systems in Asia* (2014) (http://brightergreen.org/dairy/). For more information, please visit brightergreen.org.

Introduction

Natural, Necessary, and Normal

T HE BEST FOOD THERE IS. This is what I've been told since my childhood. I drank some with every meal for a long time, and it sat proudly on the kitchen table. And whereas I often ended up leaving some food on my plate, I always emptied my glass. I would even ask for more. With its immaculate color and creamy coolness, how could you fail to find it comforting? Milk, since it's milk we're talking about, doesn't even need to be named to evoke childhood, abundance, and purity. It is, after all, our first food. Isn't it nature's superfood, too? Which is lucky, since milk is everywhere: in grilled-cheese sandwiches, frozen yogurts, and milk cartons at schools; in government health recommendations; at the heart of our economy: it is our very bread and butter.

I still remember Mr. Sealtest. That wasn't his real name. But it was the one written on his truck, spelled in white letters against a red background. Every two days, my mother would place a small card in our kitchen window. For me, it symbolized a promise of happiness. For Mr. Sealtest, it was a sign of our order: a few bags of milk and occasionally some ice cream. I still remember the way he'd say "Hello," his melancholy smile, the small talk about weather that defied the forecasts, vacations that were slow in coming. At the time, if someone had asked me where milk came from, my answer would unhesitatingly have been, "From Mr. Sealtest's truck" (of course, I knew it also came from the grocery store, but theirs was not as good). I loved Mr. Sealtest. I loved milk.

Today, I feel as if I used to live in *The Truman Show*. In this film, Truman Burbank, played by Jim Carrey, is unknowingly the star of a reality show. He lives in a small model town where flowerbeds are elegant and neighbors always courteous. In reality, his neighbors are actors and the city, a film set. When he discovers the deception, Truman is completely disillusioned.

As in *The Truman Show*, my love endured for a long time. And I too ended up completely disillusioned. I saw that I'd had it all wrong the moment I realized that milk is not essential for good health, but rather that certain nutrients are. The proof? Seventy-five percent of all humans cannot digest milk. But if drinking milk is not essential, then raising hundreds of thousands of suffering cows to produce it isn't either. Producing cheese, a process that emits as much CO_2 as producing meat, is just as unnecessary. The only reason to drink milk is the enjoyment it brings us. That's a high price to pay for our pleasure. Why was the truth hidden from me? Like Truman, I too felt I'd been duped. I felt like I'd been misled.

It is now clear to me that our relationship with milk is built on myths. Contrary to everything everyone ever told us, drinking milk is not natural, necessary, or normal. Even worse, milk consumption can lead to quite a few health problems.

To dig deeper into the problems caused by milk, I wrote *Cash Cow*, addressing ten myths about this food that most of us believe. These myths became the chapters of this book.

1. Milk Is Natural
2. A Glass of Milk for Healthy Bones
3. One Glass of Milk Is Good, but Two Is Better
4. We Can Trust the Experts
5. Schoolchildren Need Milk
6. If Cows Were Unhappy, They Wouldn't Produce Milk
7. Animal Abuse Is Illegal
8. Cheese Is Green
9. It's an Industry Just Like Any Other
10. I Could Never Live Without Cheese

Weaning Ourselves off False Beliefs

Just as it's often hard to forget a high-school sweetheart, it's also not that easy to wean ourselves off our false beliefs; that is, to give up on myths. Don't we all have some desire to keep on believing?

Why are our beliefs so enduring, even after we see that they may be false? In his book *The Believing Brain*,[1] American psychologist Michael Shermer provides some valuable answers: we are more receptive to arguments that confirm our beliefs than the ones that challenge them, and we are very good at justifying our inconsistencies and believing what suits us best.

As Shermer sees it, we are also naturally gullible and open to false beliefs. Myths, religions, and magic have been used for millennia to explain reality, whereas the scientific method is only a few hundred years old. Anecdotes and old wives' tales come to mind easily, while applying science requires effort and more in-depth knowledge. Our brain is more comfortable with intuitions and emotions than with sound research based on hard evidence.

Beliefs also bring people together. Sharing a belief makes it possible to form a group and create bonds of solidarity. Birds of a feather flock together: we think the same, so we unite. This is perhaps particularly striking when it comes to religion, but this phenomenon can be seen across all social institutions. A quick browse through the discussion forums of sports team supporters, environmental activists, or moms advocating for breastfeeding will likely be enough to convince you. Which is also the reason why I found it difficult to wean myself off my own false beliefs about milk; doing so somehow made me a traitor to my Québécois identity and the community I belonged to. The liter of milk sits proudly on the checkered tablecloths of our sugar shacks.* This is what we leave out for Santa, to encourage him to take a break between chimneys. This is the treat we give children when they come home from school. It is also the cheese platter we enjoy at dinner parties with friends. In short, by giving up my false beliefs about milk, I was betraying my farmer grandfather, my mother's cooking, and my friends' warm generosity. And last but not least, I was betraying Mr. Sealtest, too.

---

*A sugar shack (or sugarhouse) is a small, usually rustic-looking building where maple sap is boiled to make maple syrup. Sugar shacks also generally serve food to the general public.

Who Are the Real Cash Cows?

According to the dictionary, a "cash cow" is a person who is exploited as a consistent and reliable source of profits. The expression originally referred to real cows used to bring in a steady supply of cash—in the form of milk. There is no doubt that dairy cows are exploited: after approximately four years of loyal service under slave-like conditions, they will all, without exception, be sent for slaughter and end up as burger meat.

However, the expression is usually used figuratively. So let's admit it—in a sense, *we* are the cash cows of the dairy industry. After many high-profile advertising campaigns and much strategic political lobbying, the industry managed to reach and retain its share of regular, satisfied customers. The economic stakes are high: in Quebec, the dairy sector is the leading agricultural industry and it's among the largest agricultural commodity industries in the United States. And although we drink less milk than we did a few years ago, we're filling our fridges with more and more cheese and yogurt.

In the past few years, I've talked a lot about the treatment of animals, marine life, and the environmental consequences of raising livestock. More often than not, people have agreed with me. Several readers have written to tell me that I have inspired them to eat less meat. But when it comes to cheese and yogurt, it's different. Dairy products are held dear.

This emotional attachment to milk is a victory for an industry we could—and ought to—challenge seriously. I am not a doctor, a nutritionist, or an animal welfare specialist, but rather a concerned citizen who is not afraid to look at studies and spend hours reading on my couch. I am hardly a shy person either: I love talking to people with greater expertise than I possess. I also love verifying and comparing information, and nitpicking for inconsistencies. And I can say with certainty that inconsistencies in our beliefs about milk abound. After having personally learned so much about milk, I needed to offer a counter-argument to the myths perpetuated by the industry. These pages contain that argument.

1

Milk Is Natural

Sure, drinking milk is natural—for babies. Our ancestors didn't drink milk. Because while all children are born with lactase—an enzyme found in our intestinal flora that allows us to digest milk—it ceases to function upon weaning. Globally speaking, adults who are able to consume milk are a minority: this trait is the result of a genetic modification that occurred in some populations seven thousand years ago. Drinking cow's milk is thus the exception to the rule. Far from being "natural," our taste for milk is primarily cultural.

I GREW UP IN A small village in Lanaudière, northeast of Montreal, where everyone knew each other. On the first day of school, there was no need to tell each other what we'd done over summer vacation. I knew everything about the lives of my classmates—just as they knew everything about mine. Until we reached second grade, the only foreigners we played with came from the next village. Their school had been closed, so they joined our already crowded classes. They came to upset our balance.

This first experience with immigrants prepared us for what came ahead: the arrival of two Vietnamese refugees—"boat people"—who, as the teacher explained to us, had fled their country and landed here without speaking a single word of French. Soon enough, they joined the normal classes. We looked at them with a mixture of admiration and curiosity. One thing was especially strange to us: they had trouble finishing their carton of milk.

I had long believed that cow's milk was "natural." By this, I mean two things: 1) that everyone drank milk; and 2) that we were designed to drink milk. In the back of my mind, there was also the idea that it must be necessary. Little did I know that only a small part of the world's population drank milk. What is "natural" for the human baby—just like any other mammal—is to drink milk from her own mother. But once weaned, humans—like all mammals—stop being able to digest milk. It is relatively exceptional, worldwide, for even one adult to succeed in doing so. My Vietnamese friends had probably never tasted cow's milk before setting foot in our class in that suburb. Perhaps every sip of it made their stomachs twist in pain. If not everyone drinks milk, it stands to reason that it cannot be necessary.

To understand this, we have to go back to Biology 101. It all starts with enzymes. Like armies of workers, each with their own specific task, enzymes take action on the very structure of our body—like with keratin, which produces our hair—or play the role of catalysts in certain biochemical reactions, causing or accelerating these reactions. In particular, they help transform the foods we ingest so that they can be absorbed by the body.

It is in fact one of these digestive enzymes—lactase—that enables us to digest milk. It is active during the first few years of life, especially in breastfed babies. More specifically, lactase converts one of the carbohydrates in milk—lactose—into galactose and glucose, two sugars the body uses as energy. But, for reasons still unknown, as children grow, the activity of the enzyme decreases. This is a general rule of human biology.

What about the exception? Occasionally, the gene responsible for lactase production mutates. In the different populations studied, researchers have identified three genetic mutations. Because of these mutations, some people maintain their ability to digest milk in adulthood. This phenomenon is called "lactase persistence."

The Flintstones Did Not Drink Milk

Fred and Wilma Flintstone did not drink milk. In the Stone Age, there was no agriculture and animals—with the exception of Dino—had not yet been tamed. Of course, the Flintstones are not a highly reliable source when it comes to prehistory, but one thing is certain: we haven't been drinking cow's milk forever.

In fact, milk consumption became possible with the advent of agriculture and animal domestication a little over ten thousand years ago. Back in those days, our *Homo sapiens* ancestors had already shared our physiology for thousands of generations. The Lascaux Cave paintings, some seventeen thousand years old, were already ancient history by then, for instance. Before humans domesticated animals, there was not one drop of milk in our diet. This is easy enough to

understand—it is simply not possible to milk wild animals.*
The history of milk as a food is therefore intimately linked
to the history of taming mammals who can potentially be
milked: cows, sheep, goats, camels, donkeys, and even horses.

Wolves were the first animals domesticated by man—
they became domestic dogs.[1] As they increasingly founded
settlements, our ancestors are believed to have gone on to
tame pigs, goats, and sheep. As for cows, their ancestors are
aurochs, enormous wild cattle that were domesticated some
ten and a half thousand years ago.[2] These aurochs were first
used for plowing and meat. Only gradually did we begin
consuming their milk. Thus, although traces of milk are
found in Anatolian pottery that is nine thousand years old,[3]
the systematic practice of milking cattle would only begin
two thousand years later. It is thought that we first used milk
to make cheese and butter, which are easier to digest than
fresh milk.

Lactase, the Enzyme for Milk Digestion

It is believed, however, that the persistence of the enzyme
lactase, which allows adults to digest milk, appeared about
seven thousand years ago in the Fertile Crescent (now
occupied by Lebanon, Cyprus, Kuwait, Israel, Palestine,
parts of Jordan, Syria, Iraq, Iran, Egypt, and southeastern
Turkey).[4] This genetic mutation is believed to have then
spread elsewhere around the world.

Until the 1960s, the idea that virtually all adults
produce lactase was widely accepted in North America.[5] An

---

* It is very likely, however, that hunters tasted the milk of dead animals.

undeniably ethnocentric point of view! We now know that we were wrong. It is primarily populations whose ancestors hail from Europe or from nomadic African peoples who can digest milk in adulthood. In fact, a mere 25 percent of the global population exhibits lactase persistence.[6]

In northern countries, both in Europe and America, up to 80 percent of people can digest milk. But this percentage drops as we travel south. In Greece and Italy, only five percent of adults have the enzyme. Elsewhere in the world, disparities are huge. In Africa, for example, some populations exhibit a hundred percent lactase persistence, while it is completely absent in other, sometimes neighboring, populations. In Asia, the ability to digest lactose is generally non-existent, with the exception of some areas of the Middle East and India.[7]

Given the effect milk has on the digestive system of the lactose-intolerant (that is to say, three-quarters of the human population) its reputation as a "purgative" is no coincidence. Cultures that do not consume milk sometimes consider it a "dirty" fluid, much like urine.[8] I will address the symptoms of lactose intolerance (not to be confused with a milk allergy) in Chapter 3.

We Are Not All Created Equal

Most experts agree that the ability to digest milk in adulthood has probably increased over time, at least in some regions of the world. That's because this change is an adaptive advantage. In Africa, there is a fairly strong correlation between having ancestors who were livestock breeders and exhibiting lactase persistence. For these breeders, the ability to digest lactase brought nutritional benefits: milk is indeed a source of protein and fat that is available year-round. This new ability is also thought to have contributed to the successful transition from a lifestyle based on hunting to an agrarian one: indeed, by consuming both the milk and meat of an animal, you get far more calories than by consuming the meat alone.[9] It is therefore more advantageous to breed animals than to hunt them.

While there is no single explanation for the development of lactase persistence, we can find specific answers for each region of the world and each era in human history.[10]

Figure 1:1. Percentages of Lactose Intolerance in Certain Populations[11]

Vietnamese	100	Israeli Jewish	50
Thai	90	Northern Italian	50
Greek	85	French	32
Japanese	85	Caucasian American	25
African-American	70	Northern European	7
Native-American	60		

Cow's Milk Is Not Human Milk

There is one kind of milk that is truly "natural" for us to consume, and that is *human* milk. In fact, all mammals drink milk from birth to weaning. There are about five thousand four hundred species of mammals and just as many types of mammary glands. Each species is unique, as is the composition of the milk its females produce: the amounts of fat, protein, carbohydrates, sodium, etc. they contain vary according to the needs of the young.

Figure 1:2. Protein Content of Various Mammals' Milk

Milk type	Percent of protein*	Birth weight doubling time in days
Human	5	180
Horse	11	60
Cow	15	47
Goat	17	19
Dog	30	8
Cat	40	7
Rat	49	4

* Percentage of calories provided by protein. The rest comes from fat and carbohydrates.

When comparing cow's milk to human milk, one cannot help being struck by the dissimilarities. Calves seem to need almost four times more protein and calcium than human babies, which is not that surprising, given that a calf doubles its birth weight in forty-seven days, while a child needs about six months.[12]

The Lactation Station

Could an adult human drink breast milk? Jess Dobkin, a Toronto artist, has addressed this issue by creating a performance art piece entitled *Lactation Station*, a rather disturbing project in which the public is invited to sample milk from our own species. Just like in wine tastings, the artist describes each milk, giving a few details about the woman who produced it and her diet. Then, the white liquid is served in small plastic cups for people to taste.

I attended Dobkin's performance in Montreal in the spring of 2012. It took some courage. I will admit that the idea of drinking breast milk disgusted me. Yet the milk offered to us was in no way dangerous—it had even been pasteurized. I went for it. The first thing I noticed was that the taste was strong, really strong. It was definitely a long way from the neutral flavors of the grocery-store milk to which we are accustomed. My second impression was that it was sweet, sickly so. I struggled to finish my three sips. I had clearly been weaned!

Likes, Dislikes, and Perceptions

We drink cow's milk and eat goat's and sheep's cheese, but the very idea of drinking human milk—or milk from a mare or a dog—is repugnant to us. Why? It's all a matter of perception. We perceive foods as good or bad, energizing or sophisticated, pure or impure. These perceptions, which are often culturally acquired, explain why a Hindu finds it disgusting to eat beef, and why a Westerner is reluctant to ingest dog or cat meat.

Our perceptions are structured by what psychologists call schema and mental categories. These are psychological frameworks that automatically organize and interpret information we receive.[13] For example, the word "doctor" probably conjures up the image of a man in a white coat with a stethoscope around his neck who receives patients at his office or a hospital. Even though a large number of doctors are women, or work in different environments, we perceive doctors through this schema and these mental categories.

We also happen to have mental categories for the animals we see around us: the ones we eat and the ones we love,

Figure 1:3. Nutrients per 100 Grams of Milk (in Grams)

	Protein	Carbo-hydrates	Sodium	Phosphorus	Calcium
Human	1.1	9	16	18	33
Cow	4	4.9	50	97	118

the ones that produce milk for humans and the ones that produce milk for their own offspring. That is why, when we have a glass of milk in front of us, we will see a nourishing white drink rather than a warm liquid that comes from the udder of a cow—and is intended for a calf.*

Psychologist Melanie Joy wonders whether the absence of disgust that allows us to drink cow's milk or eat its flesh was innate or acquired. She believes it is largely acquired. We learn that it is normal to consume cow's milk and this belief protects us from experiencing a negative emotion.[14] In short, even our taste for milk is not really "natural." Ultimately, drinking cow's milk appears to be more of an exception than a rule for humans. In any case, it is far from a universal behavior: our ancestors did not drink milk, three-quarters of humanity is still lactose intolerant today, and our love for milk is acquired. However, this conclusion does not tell us anything about what we ought to do. Should we drink milk? If milk is necessary—as we are told—why is this the case?

---

* Studies indeed show that people are often uncomfortable seeing pieces of meat that resemble parts of an animal and prefer cuts that do not allow one to recognize the original shape of the living being it belonged to. The categories "foods" and "animals" are undeniably distinct.

2

A GLASS OF MILK FOR HEALTHY BONES

We don't need to drink milk to have healthy bones. Why not? Because it's far from the only dietary source of calcium. There are many plant-based alternatives that our body absorbs better. Furthermore, vitamin D and the right lifestyle habits are essential for good bone health.

IT HAPPENED ALL OF A sudden. Just about all my friends now have kids. Within a few years, the several-nights-a-week party animals transformed into the perfect parents. They seem to have learned how to comfort a baby at night instinctively. Everyone is trying to be the ideal mom or dad: loving, available, and responsible. These well-intentioned parents visit their pediatrician every year and follow all the recommendations made by health care professionals and found in the guide *From Tiny Tot to Toddler*[1] that was provided to them. In this thick four-color brochure, the message is clear: children must drink milk—lots of milk. A friend told me that the pediatrician suggested giving his four-year-old son 25 to 34 oz. per day. Another showed me a list of tips a nurse had given her to encourage her daughter to drink milk:

- offer small amounts of milk at a time in a nice glass;
- add fruit, concentrated fruit juice, or even vanilla to milkshakes;
- chocolate milk can be a fun dessert.

I consulted doctors I know and they repeated the same thing: children must drink milk to grow and have healthy bones. As a matter of fact, don't all schools and day care centers give them dairy products? That said, as we age, we are still required to consume milk to be healthy. At each visit, my doctor reminds me that eating a little yogurt as a snack can't be bad. And then there is advertising: "One glass of milk is good, but two are better."[2] Or put more simply, "Milk: it does a body good."[3]

Milk Has No Miraculous Properties

In fact, come to think of it, isn't it a little bit strange that a weaned, adult human being should *have* to drink the milk of another mammal to have strong bones and be healthy? This would be an exception in nature: no other animal drinks another species' milk. Our closest cousin, the chimpanzee, with whom we share 99 percent of our genetic code,[4] does not drink a single drop of milk once weaned at the age of three or four years. And yet chimpanzees don't suffer from osteoporosis—and neither do the majority of humans who are lactose intolerant.

Children are the largest consumers of milk. A healthy child is a child with a milk carton in hand; a school that failed to give milk to its students would be a bad school. Yet there is no evidence that drinking milk during childhood helps build a better skeleton. A team of researchers analyzed the results of fifty-eight studies on the link between milk consumption and bone health. Their findings, published in 2005 in the journal *Pediatrics*, are undeniable: "[I]n clinical, longitudinal, retrospective, and cross-sectional studies, neither increased consumption of dairy products, specifically, nor total dietary calcium consumption has shown even a modestly consistent benefit for child or young adult bone health. Scant evidence supports nutrition guidelines focused specifically on increasing milk or other

What Is Osteoporosis?

Osteoporosis makes bones porous and more vulnerable to fracture from a simple fall that would normally be inconsequential.

The disease is widespread among the North American population. It affects one in four women and one in eight men.[5]

Osteoporosis is not a virus or bacteria that you can catch. It is an imbalance between bone formation and bone resorption. Bone loss is the result of many factors, including genetics, diet, physical activity, and hormone production. Menopausal women are more likely to develop osteoporosis than men. This may be explained by a rapid decrease in estrogen production, which would affect the production and quality of existing collagen fibers, and therefore the skeleton as well.

dairy product intake for promoting child and adolescent bone mineralization."[6]

Adults who do have bone density loss or osteoporosis did not acquire these conditions because of insufficient milk intake. There are many potential causes including hereditary factors and lifestyle habits.

Calcium on Your Plate

Although it is not necessary to drink milk to have healthy bones, we do need calcium. However, experts struggle to agree on the exact amount of calcium we should consume. While the World Health Organization and the United Nations Food and Agriculture Organization (FAO) recommend a minimum intake of 400 mg to 500 mg per day to prevent osteoporosis,[7] in North America, official recommendations for calcium intake are 1,000 mg for people between nineteen and fifty years of age.[8] It seems that the more risk factors the target population has (consumption of coffee, salt, tobacco, lack of physical activity, low sun exposure), the higher the calcium recommendations are.

But most importantly, it should be noted that milk is by no means the only dietary source of calcium. There are many others. Figure 2:1 on pages 21 to 23 compares the amounts of calcium in different foods.[9]

What Matters Is the Bioavailability

The bioavailability of a nutrient is the proportion that the body can actually utilize in relation to the amount absorbed. The calcium found in many plants has greater bioavailability than the calcium in milk. On average, we absorb 30 percent

The Misleading Calcium Paradox

It was long believed that the consumption of animal protein could exacerbate bone decalcification. The idea was that animal protein, unlike plant protein, increased blood acidity. In the highly publicized *China Study*[10] (published in 2004), Drs. T. Colin and Thomas M. Campbell even spoke of the "calcium paradox." Greater hip fracture rates had been observed in developed countries, where calcium intake is high, compared to other countries with lower calcium intakes. The high consumption of animal protein in industrialized countries seemed to explain the phenomenon: it was believed to decalcify bones.

The American biochemist and physician reviewed ten studies together and found that when the intake of animal protein increased, the amount of calcium found in urine also increased.[11] They noted that the countries with the highest animal protein consumption were the same ones with the most fractures.[12]

These results would have served my purpose quite well! But recent studies have shed new light on this "calcium paradox."[13–15] In fact, meat increases the amount of calcium absorbed. The calcium excreted in urine is thus not calcium drawn from bones, but a surplus. As for fractures in countries where calcium intake is high, they are thought to be related to lifestyle. Dr. Michael Greger, a vegan doctor who gives dozens of lectures on nutrition each year, decided to stop talking about decalcification caused by protein: "Frankly I was convinced back then, but this new study [. . .] puts the nail in the coffin [of the calcium paradox]."[16]

But we should not conclude that this means animal protein is good for health or essential for calcium absorption. The idea is only to question the widely held view that the consumption of meat is linked to osteoporosis.

of the calcium found in dairy products and fortified foods (orange juice, tofu, soymilk) and twice that amount when it comes to the calcium found in some green vegetables like bok choy, broccoli, and kale.[17]

Figure 2:1. Calcium in Different Foods

Foods	Portion	Calcium (mg)
Vegetables		
Collard greens, frozen, cooked	½ cup (125 ml)	189
Spinach, frozen, cooked	½ cup (125 ml)	154
Collard greens, cooked	½ cup (125 ml)	141
Turnip greens, frozen, cooked	½ cup (125 ml)	132
Spinach, cooked	½ cup (125 ml)	129

Turnip greens, cooked	½ cup (125 ml)	104
Kale, frozen, cooked	½ cup (125 ml)	95
Fruits		
Orange juice, calcium-enriched	½ cup (125 ml)	155
Milk and Milk Substitutes		
Buttermilk	1 cup (250 ml)	370
Goat milk, enriched	1 cup (250 ml)	345
Soy or rice beverage, calcium-enriched	1 cup (250 ml)	319–324
Milk, homogenized 3.3%, 2%, 1%, skim, chocolate	1 cup (250 ml)	291–322
Powdered milk	4 Tbsp (24 g) of powder will yield 1 cup (250 ml) of milk	302
Cheese		
Gruyère, Swiss, goat, low-fat Cheddar, low-fat Mozzarella	1½ oz (50 g)	396–506
Processed cheese (Cheddar, Swiss, or low-fat Cheddar), sliced	1½ oz (50 g)	276–386
Cheddar, Colby, Edam, Gouda, Mozzarella, Blue	1½ oz (50 g)	252–366
Ricotta	1½ oz (50 g)	269–356
Cottage	1 cup (250 ml)	146–217

Other		
Yogurt, plain	¾ cup (175 g)	292–332
Yogurt, fruit on the bottom	¾ cup (175 g)	221–291
Soy yogurt	¾ cup (175 g)	206
Drinkable yogurt	6.75 oz (200 ml)	190
Kefir	¾ cup (175 g)	187
Fish and Seafood		
Sardines, Atlantic, canned, in oil	2½ oz (75 g)	286
Salmon (pink, red/sockeye), canned, with bones	2½ oz (75 g)	179–208
Mackerel, canned	2½ oz (75 g)	181
Sardines, Pacific, canned, with tomato sauce, with bones	2½ oz (75 g)	180
Anchovies, canned	2½ oz (75 g)	174
Meat Substitutes		
Tofu, made with calcium sulfate	¾ cup (150 g)	243–347
Beans (Navy, white), canned or cooked	¾ cup (175 ml)	93–141
Tahini/sesame paste	2 tbsp (30 ml)	130
Baked beans, canned	¾ cup (175 ml)	89–105
Almonds, dry-roasted, unblanched	¼ cup (60 ml)	93
Other		
Blackstrap molasses	1 tbsp (15 ml)	179

Vitamin D, the Key to Success

There is at least one point that we and dairy farmers can agree on: milk contains vitamin D, which is essential for bone health. But what they forget to mention is that this vitamin is not found in milk naturally: it is added, and has been, systematically, since the 1930s in the United States and the 1960s in Canada, to reduce the incidence of rickets.[18] We now know that vitamin D plays a key role in bone health by helping the body to absorb and use calcium. These are precisely the findings of a 2003 longitudinal meta-study performed on nurses.

One challenge associated with nutrition research is the collection of reliable data. How can we make sure, for example, that the people who say they are eating a particular food really are? A solution was found: to use subjects who were familiar with scientific and medical protocols—nurses! As a result, in 2003, researchers used data from the *Nurses' Health Study*, which had been collected since 1976.

The diets of tens of thousands of nurses were tracked to observe the correlation between hip fracture in postmenopausal women and the consumption of calcium, vitamin D, and milk. The diets of 72,337 (mostly white) menopausal women since the 1980s were closely scrutinized.[19] The conclusions are clear: increased consumption of vitamin D was associated with a lower incidence of hip fractures. However, neither milk nor calcium in the diet appears to reduce the risk of hip fracture in postmenopausal women.

Taking the Sun or a Pill

Health Canada recommends that people aged fifty and over consume three glasses of milk a day specifically to meet their vitamin D requirements,[20] as if it were the only possible source. *Canada's Food Guide* also places the same value on cheese. However, there is no vitamin D added to cheese (which therefore doesn't contain any).

The recommended amount of vitamin D has recently been revised upward to 2,000 international units (IU) per day for adults.[21] Why? Because even though milk has been fortified with vitamin D for years, most North Americans are still not getting enough of it.[22] Which is quite logical when you consider that a glass of milk contains only 120 IU.[23] This means that a person would have to drink more than fifteen glasses of milk per day to reach the recommended amount!

The best way to get enough vitamin D is exposure to the sun. From April to October, one 15-minute exposure (without sunscreen) of the hands, forearms, and face between 11 A.M. and 2 P.M., two or three times a week, is sufficient to ensure adequate intake for a healthy adult.[24] In the winter,

Milk Is Not Essential

In 2005, the British Advertising Standards Authority (the English equivalent of the Canadian Advertising Standards and the American Federal Trade Commission) forced Nestlé to withdraw a yogurt ad claiming that dairy products were essential to bone health. As the ASA saw it, the use of the word "essential" implied there was no other source of calcium, which is not true. It was therefore a case of false advertising.[25]

it is advisable for all people living in the northern parts of the U.S. and Canada (even those who drink milk!) to take a supplement.*

Them Bones Need Calcium

Since there is no miracle food for preventing osteoporosis, we must ensure that we build a good "bone stock" before we reach the age of thirty. The challenge then shifts to preventing bone loss. Here are some ways to do this:[26]

- Regular exercise, particularly the muscle-strengthening kind. Choose activities that involve high-impact, weight-bearing exercise, such as walking, running, dancing, skiing, soccer, racquet sports, or weight training;
- Vitamin D, through sun exposure or from fortified foods or supplements;
- Vitamin K, found in green leafy vegetables. A low level of vitamin K is associated with low bone density. Supplements of this vitamin appear to improve bone health;[27]
- A little less coffee and fewer soft drinks; caffeine is thought to increase calcium loss in the urine, while the phosphorus found in soft drinks is considered to negatively affect the calcium–phosphorus balance.

---

* Other sources of vitamin D are some species of fish (salmon, tuna, and trout), which should be avoided for environmental and animal-ethics reasons.

What Can We Replace Milk With?

The answer is simple: milk does not have to be replaced! If it is not essential for good health, its substitutes are not either. Milk contains no nutrients that are not found anywhere else; the vitamins and minerals in milk are also found in many plants that are neither white nor in liquid form.

So what do we find in milk? In addition to calcium and vitamin D, which I have discussed extensively, and protein, carbohydrates, and fat, milk contains phosphorus, vitamin B_2, vitamin B_{12}, selenium, pantothenic acid, and vitamin A.[28] All these nutrients are hidden in other foods that you probably already have in your pantry. For detailed descriptions of the food sources of various nutrients, visit Dieticians.ca, the website of Dieticians of Canada.

Clearly, milk does not need to be replaced, but you may want something to pour over your cereal, put in your coffee, or use in your favorite recipes. If so, there are many plant-based options. You will find several alternatives to dairy products in the Appendix, along with directions for making your own non-dairy milks. For now, here are some tips to help you find your way around the nutritional properties of the various plant-based milks sold in grocery stores:

- Fortified soy beverages are the only products with a nutritional profile similar to dairy milk, because soy is one of the few plants that contain "complete" proteins. All the nutrients of milk are found in fortified soy beverages, and in equivalent proportions. For Health Canada (and similarly for their American counterparts), dairy milk is the gold standard. This is why it recommends that people who do not drink dairy milk consume two to four servings of fortified soy beverages daily.

- Not all non-dairy beverages are fortified. If you are looking for sources of vitamin B_{12}, calcium, or vitamin D, you must read the labels. Fortified beverages should contain at least 30 percent of the recommended daily value of calcium and 45 percent of the recommended daily value of vitamin D. These figures are the same as those of cow's milk.
- Almond, rice, and flax beverages are not good sources of protein.
- Check whether your beverage is sweetened. Some flavored versions (chocolate, coffee, etc.) can contain more than 20 g of sugar per cup. Cow's milk contains about 12 grams of a natural sugar (lactose) per cup. The same amount of soy beverage contains approximately seven to eight grams of sugar. Several non-dairy milks also come in unsweetened versions.[29]

Should We Be Scared of Soy?

Of all the plant-based milks out there, soy is the most popular. But soy is also controversial. Does replacing cow's milk with soymilk mean taking unnecessary health risks? What is this soy controversy all about?

Soybeans have been grown and consumed for thousands of years in Asia.[30] However, it was not until the seventeenth century that they started to be grown in America. Today, the United States is the largest producer of soybeans, with 31 percent of the world's production, while Canada is seventh

The Protein Myth

Protein is an important nutrient because we need it to build, maintain, and repair our bodies' tissues. A variety of grains, legumes, and vegetables can provide all of the essential amino acids our bodies require. It was once thought that various plant foods had to be eaten together to get their full protein value—a practice otherwise known as protein combining or protein complementing. We now know that combining foods is not necessary to obtain all of the essential amino acids. As long as our diet contains a variety of grains, legumes, and vegetables, our protein needs are easily met.

There's no need to worry about protein, as consuming enough calories from a variety of plant-based food sources is enough to meet our protein needs.

With the traditional Western diet, the average American consumes about double the protein her or his body needs.[31]

with a little less than two percent. A soybean pod (which resembles a pea pod) contains seeds (which we refer to as "beans") from which oil is extracted—soybean oil is the top-seller worldwide after palm oil—and used as food or biofuel. What remains of the bean is then processed for animal feed. Soybean production for human consumption is thus marginal (less than seven percent). It is used to make dozens of things—not only the widely known tofu, but also miso (fermented soybean paste), tamari (traditional soy sauce), yogurt, and soy beverages. Soy "milk" is made from soaked soybeans that are ground with water and then baked.

GMOs

There are two major controversies associated with soybeans. The first surrounds the presence of genetically modified organisms (GMOs). Some 50 to 75 percent of the soybeans grown in Canada and almost 95 percent of those grown in the U.S. are genetically modified.[32,33] The effects of GMOs on human health are still poorly understood and studies conducted to date do not allow us to rule out long-term risks.[34] The fact that GMO labeling is not mandatory makes it difficult for us to know whether we're eating foods containing them. But the good news is that most soy milks and other vegan soy products are made from organically grown beans. For a soybean crop to be certified organic, the use of chemical fertilizers, pesticides, and GMO seeds is prohibited. We can therefore look for soy products with organic certification labels on them.

Isoflavones

The second controversy relates to the effects of isoflavones (or phytoestrogens) on human health. Isoflavones are natural chemicals that, once ingested, behave in the body in a similar manner to estrogen. Contrary to the popular belief that isoflavones are dangerous, many studies show that they may reduce the risk of breast cancer recurrence and offer protection against various cancers. [35–37]

In fact, large cancer organizations like the American Cancer Society and the American Institute for Cancer Research agree that two to three servings per day of whole soy foods are safe, and even healthy. Whole-soy sources include: tofu, tempeh, miso, soymilk, and edamame.[38] In other words, women with estrogen-receptor (ER) positive breast cancer may actually do even better when eating soy than avoiding it.

But can isoflavones disrupt sexual development and adversely affect male fertility? Do they have an impact on sperm count, as we often hear?[39] Most of the articles condemning soy have a common source, the Weston A. Price Foundation (WAPF), which essentially promotes raw milk and animal fats.[40] As it turns out, isoflavones do decrease sperm concentration, but not sperm count. Soy consumption is thought to be linked to larger volumes of ejaculate fluid containing the same number of sperm.[41] To date, there has not been any serious study linking soy consumption to fertility problems. As we will see in Chapter 3, men should worry more about the presence of hormones in cows' milk.

There's also this widespread myth that soy-based foods affect thyroid functions. Soy foods have no effect on thyroid function in healthy adults, even when regularly consumed for several years. People who take thyroid drugs can safely consume soy foods as long as they consistently eat about the same amount of soy each day—changes in soy intake may require small changes in thyroid medication since soy protein affects medication absorption.[42]

* * *

Yes, cow's milk is good for your bones, but only because of the nutrients it contains, and these nutrients can easily be found elsewhere without the risks associated with the consumption of dairy products.

3

ONE GLASS OF MILK IS GOOD, BUT TWO IS BETTER

Dairy products contain hormones, allergens, lactose, saturated fat, cholesterol, and pesticides, all of which—according to several studies—are linked to a surprising number of health problems.

A RE THERE ANY HEALTH PROBLEMS associated with the consumption of cow's milk? When I began my research for this book, I was pretty skeptical. I knew that not everybody drinks milk and that it's not necessary, but I never thought it could pose a threat to our health. Of course, you can always find conspiracy theories, food-poisoning stories, cases of abuse, or big corporations with the wrong ideas, but if drinking milk did jeopardize our health, you'd think we'd know, right?

Yet concerns about the effects of cow's milk on human health are not new. Even Dr. Benjamin Spock mentioned some misgivings in the 1998 edition of *Baby and Child Care*. Dr. Spock's book has long been a bible for parents. It's one of the biggest bestsellers of all time, with about 50 million copies sold since its first edition in 1946. The French version,

L'Art d'être parents, was the book my mother used the most: although over time it became worn out, some pages coming loose, she referred to it from the moment I was born until I reached my teenage years.

Dr. Spock is adamant on this point: "Cow's milk has become a point of controversy among doctors and nutritionists. There was a time when it was considered very desirable, but research has forced us to rethink this recommendation. . . . [D]airy products contribute to a surprising number of health problems."[1] And he isn't the only one to have voiced concerns. In 2001, the U.S. government asked a scientific panel to review the allegations made in milk marketing campaigns. The committee concluded that milk could not be considered a sports drink and that it didn't specifically prevent osteoporosis. But most importantly, the committee added that whole milk could play a role in the development of heart disease and prostate cancer.[2] What do Health Canada and the dairy farmers say?

No Need to Be Concerned

On their website Dairy Nutrition, Dairy Farmers of Canada make every effort to respond to the "facts and fallacies" related to dairy products. They offer a reassuring voice: "Scientific evidence supports the fact that there is no need to be concerned about the health consequences of consuming milk products." *There is no need to be concerned?* Really? Often, when someone is telling us not to worry, it's because they've got something to hide. Indeed, the marketing strategists of cigarette manufacturers are well aware of this, as evidenced by Imperial Tobacco's Project Viking report in 1986: "The ability to reassure smokers, to keep them in the franchise for as long as possible, is the focal point here."[3] As for Canada's Food Guide, it does not mention any risk related to the consumption of dairy products.

I tried to understand what the actual situation was. I read dozens of scientific studies and compared different sources. What I read left me both surprised and terrified. The glass of cow's milk that is supposed to keep us healthy seems to actually be one of the causes of the most common diseases in our society. So what does cow's milk contain that we should be worried about?

Milk Contains Hormones

Milk producers assure us there are no hormones in cow's

Figure 3:1. Lactation Curve of Dairy Cows

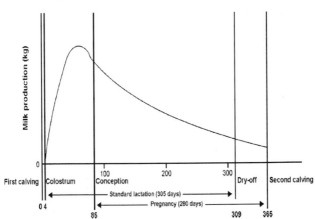

Timothy Simalenga and R. Anne Pearson, *Using Cows for Work*, University of Edinburgh, 2003[4]

milk sold in Canada. This is partly true. Artificial growth hormones—such as recombinant bovine somatotropin (rBST) used in the U.S. to increase dairy cows' milk production—are not allowed in Canada.* But this doesn't mean no hormones are found in milk at all. On the contrary, milk contains a significant number: pregnancy hormones produced by cows and growth hormones to help their calves grow.

For a cow to give milk, she must first give birth to a calf. The gestation period lasts nine months and, in nature, a cow would nurse her baby from six to nine months before becoming pregnant again. Nowadays, dairy cows continue to produce milk while they are pregnant. In fact, "modern" cows are milked three hundred and five days per year, which means they are also milked during most of their pregnancy. Eighty percent of the milk produced therefore comes from pregnant cows. And that's why it contains a significant concentration of estrogen and progesterone, two pregnancy hormones.

The Lactation Cycle of Cows
Milk also contains natural growth hormones, IGF-1

---

* rBST is a genetically modified artificial growth hormone given to dairy cows by injection. It's unclear whether the hormone poses health risks to humans. Although there is no definitive proof that the use of rBST leads to breast and other cancers, there is now enough evidence to take precautionary measures and to eliminate its use. Because of the potential human health impacts of using rBST, U.S. consumers have successfully persuaded many companies to switch to rBST-free milk. Major U.S. grocery chains Kroger, Safeway, and Walmart now prohibit the use of rBST in their store-brand milk products. rBST is also known as rBGH (recombinant bovine growth hormone).

(insulin-like growth factor). In both cows and humans, IGF-1 is secreted mainly by the liver and released into the blood. These hormones play a large role in the growth of children, and they also have effects on muscle development in adults. IGF-1 hormones are naturally found in milk to promote growth in human babies and calves. Whereas the cow's milk produced in the United States contains a greater concentration of IGF-1 because American cows are given additional growth hormones, cow's milk produced in Canada also contains some since these naturally occurring IGF-1 hormones are not destroyed by pasteurization (the process in which milk is heated to kill bacteria).[5]

Cow Hormones in the Human Body

So, we know there are hormones in the cow's milk we consume. But are they absorbed? And if so, do we absorb enough of them for there to be an effect on our bodies? Recent studies say yes to both questions.[6] In 2009, Kazumi Maruyama's team of Japanese researchers measured the concentration of estrogen and progesterone in the serum and urine of young men and prepubescent children after they drank milk. They also examined the effect of daily consumption of milk on the menstrual cycle of healthy women. When cow's milk contains a high concentration of estrogen and progesterone, the time of ovulation can be affected.[7]*

After drinking milk, testosterone levels decreased in men and the blood concentration of pregnancy hormones (estrogen and progesterone) significantly increased in

---

* Like their Canadian counterparts, Japanese cows do not receive rBST treatments.

women—enough to reach a level that can be associated with an increased risk of multiple ovulations. Moreover, high milk consumption is linked to twin pregnancies: women who drink milk are five times more likely to give birth to twins than those who don't consume any.[8]

Health Impacts

It is difficult to determine the true effects of cow hormones on human health. Control studies are impossible, since all cow's milk contains them. (Even consumers of organic milk are ingesting pregnancy and growth hormones.) The absorption of pregnancy hormones throughout one's life may have consequences, and more and more researchers are convinced that our system cannot handle this invasion of cow hormones. They are thought to be partly responsible for the development of acne and certain cancers.

Acne is a nightmare for teenagers. Genetic predisposition, stress, perspiration, and certain medications play a role in its development. But while it affects up to 85 percent of Western teenagers, it is nonexistent in populations that don't consume milk.[9] Although the causal link is difficult to establish, the concentration of hormones in cow's milk is high enough to stimulate sebum production. IGF-1, in particular, may be involved. The natural production of IGF in our bodies peaks at around the age of fifteen. Adding IGF from cow's milk could amount to fanning the flames.[10] Female milk drinkers also seem to suffer from more acne than women who do not drink milk. A large study involving 47,000 women found that those who consumed the most milk were more prone to acne as teens.[11] Published in 2006, another study on 6,094 girls from nine to fifteen years of age confirmed that the girls who drank the most cow's milk were the most acne-prone.[12] The link between milk consumption and the development of cancer is more difficult to establish. Since the 1960s, a significant increase in the number of cases of estrogen-related diseases—such as ovarian, uterine, testicular, and prostate cancers—has nonetheless been observed. And in the search for correlations between these cancers and eating habits, the one thing that stands out is the high prevalence of milk and cheese in patients' diets. But what has changed in our milk since the 1960s? The fact that cows are now lactating while pregnant, and therefore the increase of the hormone levels found in milk.[13–15] The concentration of hormones in milk may also put women who drink large amounts of it after menopause at an increased risk of breast cancer.[16] Indeed, estrogen plays a role in cell proliferation and could thus promote the growth of cancer cells. At the same time, evidence from large prospective cohort studies and meta-analyses suggests a protective role for milk and milk products in colorectal cancer. It is not clear whether it's the milk itself or calcium that plays this role.[17]

Nevertheless, Harvard researchers studied the profiles of 100,000 women aged twenty-six to forty-six. Those with the highest intake of meat and dairy products also had the highest risk of breast cancer (33 percent more than those who consumed the least).[18] In a 2006 meta-study, scientists who analyzed the primary data of twelve studies on the subject found an increased risk of ovarian cancer in women drinking three glasses of milk or more per day.[19] And men are not exempt: over twenty studies establish a link between prostate cancer and cow's milk consumption.[20] The best way men can fight this cancer may be to shave their milk mustaches!

Finally, several studies show a link between the absorption of IGF-1 and cancer. An explanatory hypothesis is that hormones could increase the risk of developing the disease by preventing malignant cells from dying.[21]

Milk Contains Allergens

We imagine that someone with food allergies never leaves home without their EpiPen and that they run the risk of dying if they come into contact with those specific allergens—usually nuts. But it's also possible to suffer from allergies for years without knowing it. In fact, the symptoms of a food allergy—chronic fatigue, anxiety, heart palpitations, etc.—can prove difficult to identify. Recent epidemiological studies suggest that nearly four percent of Americans are afflicted with food allergies.[22] The allergy to cow's milk is one of the most common. Official figures speak of 0.3 percent of Canadians,[23] but it could affect 7.5 percent of the Canadian population.[24] In children, it is the most common allergy.[25]*

Allergic reactions are triggered when mast cells come into contact with the allergen. The one that is largely responsible for a milk allergy is beta-casein, a protein. When mast cells come into contact with beta-casein, they release histamines, molecules that stimulate mucus production, muscle contraction, and inflammation.[26]

---

* Other commonly found allergens are gluten, corn, citrus, egg white, and soy.

Symptoms Associated with a Milk Allergy

The following scene happened in the cafeteria of an office, and similar situations undoubtedly arise again and again in our Western culture. For dessert after her lunch, my then-very-pregnant friend Julie bites into an apple. Immediately, as if to avert a disaster, a co-worker turns to her and says, "You don't eat yogurt? But you had no dairy in your lunch. Think of your baby!" Everyone seems to believe that we need to consume dairy products during pregnancy. But this belief is unfounded. Recent studies show that vegan mothers (who do not consume any dairy products) eating a balanced diet give birth to healthy children.[27]

In reality, rather than putting their baby's health at risk, women who avoid dairy products before, during, and after pregnancy actually reduce their children's risk of the adverse side effects of milk consumption, including type 1 diabetes, ear infections, iron deficiency, and colic.[28–31] These problems are often symptoms associated with an allergic reaction—most often to cow's milk.

But adults too can suffer from milk allergies. Indeed, cow's milk contains at least thirty proteins that can cause allergic reactions. These can be immediate or appear twenty-four to seventy-two hours later. Symptoms may last from several days to several weeks.[32] And since the reaction is not always instantaneous, it is possible to be allergic to milk for years without knowing it.

Headaches and asthma seem to be two common symptoms. For example, after removing all dairy products from the diets of forty-eight patients suffering from either migraine or asthma, thirty-three of them saw their condition improve significantly.[33] A recent study confirmed that ear infections can also be caused by a milk allergy.[34] Indeed, the body reacts to the allergen by producing mucus, fluids, and inflammation in the throat, nose, and ear tubes, which creates the ideal breeding ground for bacteria—and ear infection. In a 1994 study, food allergens were removed from the diets of one hundred and four children suffering from ear infections. In 86 percent of the cases, the infection cleared. For most, the allergen responsible for the problem was cow's milk.[35]

Similarly, arthritis and joint pain often come from a milk allergy. There are many testimonials from people who have overcome their condition by cutting out dairy products. Thousands of Quebecers have read Jacqueline Lagacé's story *Comment j'ai vaincu la douleur chronique par l'alimentation* (*The End of Pain* in English). In her book, she reports that in under eighteen months she regained the use of her fingers by removing gluten, dairy, and other allergens from her diet.

A similar case was reported in the *British Medical Journal* in the 1980s.[36] A thirty-eight-year-old woman was suffering from severe arthritis and no medication had been successful in relieving her pain. A doctor noticed that she was consuming a lot of cheese—up to one pound per day—and suggested that she eliminate all dairy products. In less than two weeks, the symptoms of her arthritis began to disappear. After a few months, she had almost fully recovered and wasn't taking any medication. To test his hypothesis, the doctor asked her to reintroduce cheese into her diet. Less than twenty-four hours later, the pain was back. The symptoms then disappeared again when she stopped consuming dairy products.

Like arthritis, type 1 diabetes is an autoimmune disease—that is to say, the body attacks itself. It occurs most often in children and adolescents, which is why it is also called juvenile diabetes. The pancreas of diabetics is unable to produce insulin, which converts glucose, or blood sugar. Since a diabetic's body does not produce insulin, the sugar level in the blood increases dangerously.

The causes of this type of diabetes are still not well understood. But in 1999, some researchers hypothesized that it was linked to an allergic reaction to milk. They presented their results at a major conference of the American Diabetes Association.[37] Since then, around one hundred studies that confirm their findings have been published on the subject.[38] When examining the data by country, we find a strong correlation between the incidence of type 1 diabetes and the amount of milk consumed by children.[39] The younger they are exposed to cow's milk, the greater the risk of developing an autoimmune reaction that can cause diabetes.

And finally, one last important thing to know is that the most frequent source of colic in infants is an allergy to cow's milk. Unfortunately, breastfed children are not immune to this problem since their mother can pass the cow's milk protein on to them through their own milk.[40,41] Maybe a fussy baby is just trying to say that they're allergic to their mom's yogurt.

Milk Contains Lactose

Many people confuse a milk allergy to milk intolerance. As we have seen, the allergy is caused by certain proteins and triggers immune reactions, while intolerance results from the lack of lactase, an enzyme that helps digest milk. Three-quarters of the human population is thought to be lactose intolerant (for more on this, see Chapter 1).

When someone who doesn't produce lactase consumes milk, gastrointestinal symptoms appear between thirty minutes and two hours after ingestion: bloating, diarrhea, abdominal pain, or cramps, vomiting (especially in children), and constipation.

Lactose content varies from one dairy product to another. Due to the processing milk undergoes to become cheese, it is easier for adults to absorb milk in cheese form, even when they do not produce lactase.

Figure 3:2. Lactose Amounts

	Amount of lactose[42]
Yogurt (1 cup)	16 g
Fluid milk (1 cup)	13.02 g
Cheddar cheese (50 g)	0.12 g

Milk Contains Saturated Fat and Cholesterol

If there is one nutrition issue today on which scientific consensus does exist, it is that the two most significant risk factors for heart disease are saturated fat intake and cholesterol. And cow's milk contains both. For example, a one-cup glass of 2% milk contains 3.3 g of saturated fat and 21 mg of cholesterol, and a 50-g piece of cheddar cheese has 10.5 g of saturated fat and 53 mg of cholesterol.[43] Even the U.S. Food and Drug Administration agrees: "Some fats are more likely to cause heart disease. . . . These fats are usually found in foods from animals, such as meat, milk, cheese, and butter."[44]

However, the correlation between dairy consumption and the risk of developing coronary heart disease is difficult to establish, and many studies find conflicting results.[45] A recent article published by American Heart Association journals shows that dairy products with a high fat content are associated with an increased risk of coronary heart disease in women.[46] Women at risk should therefore be cautious.

Even 2% milk is a significant source of fat. By weight, it is true that only two percent of the liter of milk is made up of lipids. But it's the proportion of calories from fat that must be measured to compare the fat content of different foods: if we take a pat of butter and mix it with one quart of water, the proportion of fat in the jug will be less than if the same amount of butter is mixed with one cup of water. However, the total amount of fat remains the same. What you want to measure is the number of calories in what you eat that come from fat. In a glass of 2% milk, 34 percent of the calories come from fat, while Health Canada recommends limiting the proportion of calories from fat to 20 to 35 percent in adults.[47] In other words, even milk with two percent fat is very rich. But nothing beats cheese: in your average cheese, 70 percent of calories come from fat, especially saturated fat—the kind that blocks arteries.

Oddly enough, the industry invests significant resources in trying to convince us that dairy products are essential to maintaining a healthy weight. In the United States, the National Dairy Council has spent $200 million over two years to promote the idea that cow's milk facilitates weight loss.[48] In Canada, dairy producers have even created a website dedicated to this topic: yourhealthyweight.ca. Yet independent studies do not link weight loss and consumption of dairy products.[49,50] They even tend to show the reverse trend. The U.S. milk producers' campaign correlating milk consumption and weight loss had to be withdrawn due to lack of scientific evidence.[51]

Noting that few studies had been conducted over long periods, researchers monitored a group of nearly 13,000 American children for three years, between 1996 and 1999. They documented the changes in their body mass. Children who drank the most milk also put on the most weight. The researchers were clear about the study's results: "Our findings did not support theories that greater milk intake will contribute to the control of overweight."[52]

Milk Contains Casomorphins

Sudden infant death syndrome (SIDS) is the leading cause of death for infants between one month and one year of age.[53] The identified risk factors are sleep position, secondhand smoke, and an overheated room. However, casomorphins produced by the breakdown of the casein in the cow's milk consumed by the mother and passed on to her child through her breast milk also seem to be involved.

Casomorphins are peptides, or protein fragments, the effects of which on the nervous system are similar to that of morphine, which is why babies often fall asleep while nursing. In a young child with a nervous system that is not yet fully developed, casomorphins could hinder the part of the brain responsible for breathing, thus causing apnea (respiratory arrest) or death. The phenomenon is rare because, in general, an enzyme breaks down casomorphins. But in some infants, this enzyme does not function properly.[54,55] Infants who drink (or whose mothers consume) cow's milk are twice as likely to suffer from sudden infant death syndrome as those who don't.[56]

Milk Contains Pesticides

Cow's milk may also be linked to the development of Parkinson's disease. A study conducted on 7,500 men showed that those who drank more than two glasses of milk per day were twice as likely to contract the disease as those who didn't consume any milk.[57] Another study analyzed the cases of 57,000 men and 73,000 women over nine years. The link between milk consumption and the development of the disease was striking in men, but non-existent in women. While all dairy products increased the risk of suffering from Parkinson's disease, it is the correlation with milk consumption that seemed the strongest. The underlying mechanism, however, remains unclear.[58] Some researchers suggested that the cause might lie not in the nutrients in milk, but in the pesticides that pass from what the cow eats into the milk it produces.[59]

* * *

I will now stop this tedious and daunting—but necessary—list of the components of milk that seem to have undesirable effects. Needless to say, we shouldn't conclude from the

The Devil Is in the Details

In his book *Devil in the Milk*,[60] New Zealand professor of agriculture Keith Woodford explains how beta-casein (a milk protein) varies with cow genetics. He describes the two major beta-casein families: A1 and A2. There are therefore two kinds of cows: A1 and A2. Why is this an important detail? Because the beta-casein of the A1 family is believed to release an opiate called BCM-7 when we digest it. No such opiate is released from A2 cow's milk. This opiate from the A1 cows may be responsible for the many ills I have just described: heart disease, type 1 diabetes, and autoimmune diseases.

For the time being, it is impossible to find A2 milk in North America. It is however common in Europe, Australia, and New Zealand. The author advocates replacing herds of A1 cows with cows from the A2 type. This idea is still controversial and we will have to follow relevant developments in the coming years.

above that milk is poison. Even if a given substance presents potential hazards, it doesn't mean that we should avoid consuming it. We have, however, seen that we don't need milk to be healthy. Not only is cow's milk not necessary, but we now know that its consumption can be harmful to human health. Perhaps drinking milk is taking an unnecessary risk. Conversely, cutting milk out of our diet could relieve us of many symptoms. So why aren't doctors suggesting it?

Let Thy Food Be Thy Medicine

Born in 460 BCE, Hippocrates, the father of medicine, is said to have spoken of the importance of a healthy diet for healthy living with these words: "Let thy food be thy medicine." The problem is that those who take his oath today base their practice on medication and surgery. Nutrition is still only rarely taught in medical schools—during their four years of training, aspiring doctors will often take no nutrition courses at all.[61]

Despite the success of books like *Foods That Fight Cancer: Preventing Cancer through Diet* by Drs. Richard Béliveau and Denis Gingras (McClelland & Stewart, 2006) or *Anticancer: A New Way of Life* by David Servan-Schreiber (Viking, 2008), our society still treats the sick with medication, not food. Yet 70 percent of all chronic degenerative diseases are linked to diet and could therefore be prevented.[62] In medicine, the expression "Tomato Effect" is used to refer to rejection of an effective treatment for absurd reasons. Until the nineteenth century, Americans refused to eat tomatoes because they believed they were poisonous. Everyone *knew* they were toxic and nobody questioned that belief, until one day someone ate some tomatoes and survived. Similarly, many treatments have been rejected by the medical profession based only on the belief that they wouldn't work. This suggests that doctors may dismiss the idea that the consumption of dairy products could cause a disease simply because it seems impossible to them.[63]

It should also be pointed out that it isn't vegetable producers that are funding research—it's mainly the pharmaceutical industry. Dr. Alain Vadeboncoeur, vice-president of Quebec Doctors for Medicare, feels that the State's withdrawal in the matter "leaves the door wide open to the private sector in strategic areas such as scientific research or continuing education for physicians."[64] It is quite possible that you now know much more than your doctor about the role of cow's milk in a balanced diet and its effects on health. It isn't bad faith on the part of doctors; it's just that no one has given them the information. That being said, who would agree to leave a medical clinic with a crying baby suffering from an ear infection with no prescription other than to cut out cow's milk "to see what happens"? I know several people who would rush to see another doctor, one who prescribes "real" treatments.

Finally, it is important to keep in mind that even the best-intentioned health specialists often cannot help being swayed by the millions of dollars spent on advertising. In the absence of specific information, it is easy, even for a doctor, to believe that milk is an essential food. Besides, this is basically what *Canada's Food Guide* and the American site *Choose My Plate* say. After all, these are supposed to be the ultimate resources for nutrition. Unfortunately, as we will see in the next chapter, there is good reason to doubt their scientific basis.

4

WE CAN TRUST THE EXPERTS

Official nutrition guidelines and dairy producers rely on data from many studies to issue their recommendation that we ought to consume dairy products daily. But these studies mysteriously yield findings different from the ones associating dairy products with health problems. How can research results end up being contradictory? The answer is influence and bias—studies funded by the industry tend to yield results that are in its interest.

I 'M NOT THE ONLY ONE trying to dispel misconceptions. Dairy Farmers of Canada is doing the same thing. The group has set up a comprehensive website that shares the most recent "scientific data" about "the potential impact of milk products in health and disease prevention."[1] It presents and then crushes any criticism, throwing around references and sentences like "The scientific evidence is insufficient to establish a causal link" or "More research is needed." Dairy Farmers of America, for its part, is more direct. The organization explains that misperceptions arise even though the beneficial role of milk products has been demonstrated.

It also cautions its readers against the pernicious effects of the Internet: "Today's multi-media environment increases opportunities for misinformation leading to misperceptions about food in general to flourish. [. . .] The Internet can contribute to consumer confusion and misperceptions about food, including dairy foods, because sites with science-based information co-exist with those containing questionable or inaccurate information from unqualified sources."[2]

Indeed, there are many websites out there publishing absolute nonsense. But it would be quite a stretch to classify Harvard researchers' publications in *The Lancet* within the non-credible source category. How is it that dairy producers' scientific studies never reach the same conclusions as those of independent researchers? Why are there no conflicting studies on topics of lower economic importance, like the effects of broccoli on our health? Could the results of some studies and the choice of policies that are implemented be influenced by the power of the dairy industry?

Revisions to the Food Guide

In Canada, the landmark text on nutrition is the *Food Guide* published by Health Canada. We all know by heart the four food groups that were listed in our school textbooks. And today, doctors and nutritionists still refer to those same groups.

In 2007, *Canada's Food Guide* was revised for the seventh time since its creation in 1942. Despite some adjustments, the guide's structure remained essentially unchanged, with its four groups: milk products, meat, grains, and fruits and vegetables. However, although we clearly do not live as our grandparents did, and science has taught us a lot about nutrition since 1940, recommendations on milk consumption haven't changed much. The biggest thing that has changed is the quantities. While in 1949 the recommendation was "a half-pint of milk a day" (or 284 ml) for adults, this amount was upped to one and a half cups (375 ml) in 1961, to finally reach two one-cup portions a day (500 ml total) from 1977 on, when the group became "milk and milk products." Today the category is called "milk and milk substitutes," and an illustration of a soy beverage carton was recently added to the guide's cover. But the impression given is that this is only a substitute for *real* milk—a plan B.*

It was probably easier for governments to advise people on what to eat during the war, a time when a large part of the population suffered from deficiencies. Today, the trend has reversed and the guide must now tell us to consume less of certain foods, but without offending anyone. There's a lot at stake. Imagine the economic consequences of a new version of the guide in which the milk products group has disappeared after being merged with meat, nuts, and legumes in a whole new group labeled "protein"!

An Independent Plate

In the United States, it is the Department of Agriculture (USDA) that is responsible for developing the food guide. Its recommendations are regularly called into question. The Harvard School of Public Health, for example, has

---

* The U.S. dietary guidelines are similar. Dairy has always been a part of the official recommendations and remains so with the most recent (2010) iteration, Choose My Plate. "Milk" became "Dairy Products" in 2010, and "fortified soy milk" was first included that same year.

Figure 4:1. The Healthy Eating Plate

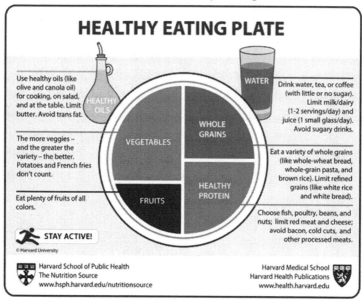

The Healthy Eating Plate," Harvard School of Public Health,
The Nutrition Source

criticized the USDA: "[The Pyramid's] blueprint was based on shaky scientific evidence, and it barely changed over the years to reflect major advances in our understanding of the connection between diet and health. [The new My Plate] still falls short on giving people the nutrition advice they need to choose the healthiest diets."[3]

In the Harvard School of Public Health's view, the USDA recommendations contain several flaws, a criticism that could also be made of *Canada's Food Guide*. For example, the official guides do not show that whole grains are a better choice than refined grains, or that beans or nuts should be preferred over red meats. The tables do not indicate the good fats. The inclusion of milk is also a problem in the eyes of the Harvard team: "Yet dairy is given a prominent place [. . .] despite evidence that high intakes of dairy products do not reduce the risk of osteoporosis and may increase the risk of some chronic diseases." For the team of scientists, the major problem in these nutritional recommendations is that they ignore much of what constitutes the standard American diet: sugary drinks, sweets, salty processed foods, refined grains, etc. In *Canada's Food Guide*, these products are classified in the "other foods" that ought to be consumed with moderation.

To address the various shortcomings of government recommendations, the Harvard researchers decided to develop their own healthy eating pyramid (which later became a plate, see Figure 4:1). First and foremost, daily exercise. Then, fruits and vegetables, whole grains, and healthy fats. Great importance is also placed on legumes. And dairy products? They suggest one to two servings a day, *or* vitamin D and calcium supplements.

Are Researchers Independent?

All recommendations on what people should eat and in what quantities are based on scientific research, whether they are issued by *Canada's Food Guide* or the information campaigns of producers. But where do these studies come from, and who subsidizes them?

It's easy to find data on milk consumption. Dairy Farmers of Canada has set up a website (dairynutrition.ca) that claims to be "the most comprehensive and up-to-date source of scientific information for the health professional on the role of milk products in nutrition and health."[4] It covers everything: the role of milk in the development of certain cancers, obesity and osteoporosis, lactose intolerance, and even the "facts and fallacies" about milk. The information is comprehensive and the sources are exhaustive.

Reading this site is a natural source of comfort. As the Quebec ad campaign says, there's no need to worry—it's natural to drink milk and it's good for your health. Any doubts you might have are immediately quelled, because conflicting studies may exist. This is the argument that the industry most frequently invokes to refute a scientific position: "Very little research shows that . . ."; "There is very little evidence to corroborate the theory that. . . ." Of course, these are not false statements. But it's not quite enough to reassure us either.

Minimizing the importance of data that contradict one's position is a strategy that has been used in the past by some interest groups. In the 1960s, when the medical profession began realizing the harmful effects of smoking and started alerting the public, the tobacco industry was quick to initiate a campaign to refute the latest research. The counter-attack strategy was pretty simple—it consisted of muddying the waters and insinuating that the situation was more complicated than it seemed. In 1968, the recommendations of Hill and Knowlton, the public relations firm of cigarette manufacturer Philip Morris, read as follows: "The most important type of story is that which casts doubt in the cause and effect theory of disease and smoking. Eye-grabbing headlines were needed and 'should strongly call out the point—Controversy! Contradiction! Other Factors! Unknowns!'"[5] Quite obviously, the tobacco industry and the dairy industry are very different, and I'm not trying to draw a parallel between the two. But they both use the same strategy: sowing the seeds of doubt.

On Dairy Farmers of Canada's site, we also learn that dairy producers financially support scientific research in Canada in the areas of nutrition, food science, and health. DFC is indeed one of the main sponsors of nutritionists' conferences and meetings, and the organization offers many training workshops to dietitians across Canada every year. We are assured that funded research is conducted impartially and remains unbiased, that the studies are selected by a committee of experts and are peer-reviewed. But can we really trust the studies cited by the dairy producers? Would they support or publish studies going against their own interests? Could "contradictory" data come from the industry?

Funded Research Favorable to the Interests of the Sponsor

Despite all the codes of ethics, industry-funded studies tend to be biased. This is what analysis of research findings in the pharmaceutical industry shows: the support from manufacturers orients the conclusions.[6] American nutritionist and scholar Marion Nestle has noted, for example, that independent studies always find a link between soft drink consumption and obesity. However, research commissioned by the soft drink industry almost never discovers this kind of connection.[7] It should be noted that the entire dairy industry is a significant funder of scientific research in health and nutrition.[8]

If researchers showed their biases, major consequences would follow, in nutrition and elsewhere. As we have seen, food guides and health professionals' recommendations are based on scientific studies, and physicians and nutritionists use the studies as well. Moreover, their findings are widely reported in the media, which directly influence people's behavior—we eat what we are told to eat! What are we to think of these biases?

Hard to say. Marion Nestle also posed this question in *Food Politics*, a fascinating book about industry influence on nutrition and health. She notes how complicated it is to find out what happens in laboratories: "I could not find *anyone* who would speak to me 'on the record' for this book. When I told friends in government, food companies, and academia that I was writing a book about how the food industry affects nutrition and health, they offered to tell me anything I wanted to know, but not for attribution."[9]

It is, therefore, unsurprising that for a long time virtually no one had dared to thoroughly and systematically study the influence of sponsors on the findings of nutrition studies. In 2007, a team of American researchers finally filled this gap. Lenard I. Lesser, formerly a physician at Boston Children's Hospital, and his colleagues analyzed the two hundred and three studies on the effects of three beverages (soft drinks, juices, and milk) published between January 1999 and December 2003.[10]

An independent group of researchers then reviewed and classified these studies' findings. The aim was to assess how the study sponsor (with interests in conflict, unrelated, or unknown) shaped the content of the conclusions (in favor of the drink, unfavorable, or neutral). What did we learn? That scientific articles funded by beverage manufacturers are four to eight times more likely to be favorable to the product than independent articles. Furthermore, no study funded by the industry reached conclusions that went against its interests!

So, industry-funded nutrition studies tend to be favorable to the sponsor. But these results do not necessarily imply that researchers tamper with data. The influence is exerted much more subtly. Lesser and his team explain the bias in favor of the sponsor's interests using the five following factors:

1. Sponsors may fund only those studies that they believe will present their products in a favorable light;

2. Investigators might formulate their hypotheses, design studies, or analyze data in ways that are consistent with the financial interests of their industrial sponsors;

Probiotic Yogurts: "Healthy"?

According to dairy-product manufacturer Dannon, the unique BL Regularis bacterial culture of its Activia yogurt "helps improve digestive comfort." In 2008, a U.S. law firm filed a class-action suit against Dannon. The prosecution alleged that the manufacturer's claims that its Activia and DanActive probiotic yogurts had been proven to "improve one's intestinal rhythm" and "regulate your digestive system" were misleading and unsubstantiated.

3. Industrial sponsors may choose to delay or not publish findings that have negative implications to the sponsor's products;

4. Authors of scientific reviews may search and interpret the literature selectively, in ways consistent with the sponsor's interests;

5. Scientific reviews arising from industry-supported scientific symposia, often published as journal supplements, may over- or under-represent certain viewpoints, if presenters whose opinions conflict with the sponsor's financial interests are not invited to participate.

Martijn B. Katan, a nutrition professor at Vrije Universiteit in The Netherlands, commented on the work of Dr. Lesser's team.[11] Katan believes that "when an industry is the major sponsor of research on its own products, unfavorable effects of that product are less likely to be investigated." This is the start of a slippery slope. Subsequently, "the dosage of the product and the nature of control treatments may be adjusted so as to increase the chances that the study will demonstrate benefits of the product or that adverse effects will not reach statistical significance." Researchers can also choose to leave unfavorable data out of the press release, or simply opt not to publish the study. Katan also points out that some contract research organizations grant the sponsor a veto on the publication of the findings.

Dairy Farmers of Canada Guidelines

Looking at the guidelines to apply for a grant from Dairy

Dannon opted for a settlement and agreed to pay $35 million to U.S. consumers who had purchased its products since their launch in 2006 and 2007. It also agreed to change its advertising.

In Canada, Dannon also settled a class-action suit brought against them in 2009 by a customer who felt that the company wrongly claimed that its products improved digestion. As a result of this settlement, Dannon announced it would make "a number of changes to its communications."[12]

Health Canada and the Canadian Food Inspection Agency (CFIA) are jointly responsible for the federal policy on food labeling governed by the Food and Drugs Act. Manufacturers do not have to submit evidence prior to developing their labels but must be able to provide supporting data upon request. Dannon detains all necessary evidence: dozens of studies have been published by its own laboratories, whereas independent research on the subject is still non-existent.[13,14]

Farmers of Canada (DFC),[15] we see some clauses suggesting that the organization has a say in the publication of the studies it funds:

- A copy of all manuscripts and/or abstracts related to a DFC-funded study should be sent to them for review and comment prior to any disclosure of findings;

- Each publication of findings from a DFC-funded study should be acknowledged in the following manner: "Supported by a Grant from Dairy Farmers of Canada," unless otherwise instructed by DFC;
- The applicant should advise DFC of forthcoming public communications of research results at conferences, symposia, media events, or the like. The applicant should acknowledge DFC's contribution to the study, unless otherwise instructed by DFC.

We also notice that research priorities are established in such a way that they can be used to promote dairy products (and reassure consumers): clarify the role of dairy products on blood pressure management; clarify the role of dairy products in bone health and prevention of osteoporosis and fractures, including the role of dairy protein; understand the reasons for under-consumption of milk products by Canadians, etc.

Dairy producers are steering the research toward topics that serve their interests and are also making sure they reserve the right of first review before publication, so that they can choose whether they want to have their name associated with certain studies.

There is no ethical problem with the dairy industry promoting milk. But we can assume that there *is* one when it sneaks into public health institutions for the sole purpose of maintaining or increasing its revenues. Meanwhile, since independent research is increasingly rare (who will fund it?),[16] it becomes almost impossible to cross-check the data released by the industry.

A Gray Area

Not everything the industry touches is unclean, and research funding by the private sector has led to significant scientific discoveries. But we must keep in mind that researchers working with dairy producers inevitably face some pressure. Although most universities have strict codes of conduct regarding relations with the industry and conflicts of interest, when the time comes to find money to keep a lab open or to financially support researchers, it may prove difficult to ensure true independence. It seems clear that nutrition research should be further subsidized by the public sector.

In my view, the crux of the problem is that milk is in a gray area. Milk is more than water and sugar. It actually contains nutrients necessary for good health, and those who say this do their jobs well. The catch is that these nutrients are also found in other foods. That's where the influence of the industry comes into play, namely when it asserts, on the basis of these studies, that we need milk to be healthy, and that we must have it in our schools!

5

SCHOOLCHILDREN NEED MILK

Marketing to children has always been central to the strategy of dairy farmers. Under the pretext of providing nutrition education, and claiming that milk is essential for good health, they encourage students to drink milk — often chocolate milk, which passes for a healthy snack even though it contains as much sugar as a soft drink. When children become adults, their interest in milk is sustained by ads appealing to their emotions.

WHEN I WAS IN ELEMENTARY school, we had nutrition class every Friday afternoon. We applied ourselves to coloring inside the lines in our big yellow activity book. We also learned to recognize the four food groups. The principles were easy to remember: chips and sodas made you fat; milk, meat, pasta, and vegetables made you grow. On the cover of that yellow book was a small cow adorned with a maple leaf—because this activity book that served as an introduction to nutrition was *courtesy of* "milk."

The rest of the week, we moved from theory to practice: every morning, we were handed a carton of milk that we drank with a straw (and it was forbidden to blow bubbles). Then we went outside for recess, full of energy and ready to test our newly solidified bones. Our energy and stronger bones were *courtesy of* "milk."

* * *

Children have always been the core of dairy producers' marketing strategy. Those in my generation—and younger people, too—remember milk cartons, while their parents remember the warm milk they were served in third-pint glass bottles.

Distributing milk in schools is hardly a new idea. In the 1920s, the Child Welfare Association was already giving cow's milk to the malnourished children of Montreal for free. A decade later, cafeterias appeared at schools. There, children could buy a half-pint of milk (284 ml) for three cents.[1]

In his article "Fattening Children or Fattening Farmers? School Milk in Britain, 1921–1941," English historian Peter Atkins explains how dairy producers took advantage of school milk programs to present it as a perfect and essential food. If all children drank milk, they would all grow properly; this would be a kind of widely distributed "insurance policy."

In the early 1930s, the depression reached the province of Quebec. Not all families could afford the luxury of a glass of milk for their children. Milk sales declined. Worried, the industry went knocking on schools' doors to offer its miracle cure for malnutrition. In 1934, the Montreal Catholic School

Commission (MCSC) met the dairy producers' demand by establishing a Catholic Social Service to be managed by a nurse, Alice Lebel, previously employed by one of the largest dairies in Montreal, J.-J. Joubert.*

It was Ms. Lebel who established the "weighing of schoolchildren." Children who were found to be underweight would be entitled to a half-pint of milk for free. The program seemed to generate results. The MCSC proudly announced that students who received free milk gained an average of 4.46 pounds.[2]

Peter Atkins reports more nuanced data. He cites studies from the 1920s and 1930s that show that milk consumption in schools grew at the expense of other protein sources. Still, in England as in Canada, school milk programs are maintained. For the National Milk and Dairy Council (the equivalent of the federation of milk producers at the time), it is a doubly winning strategy: first, it boosts sales, and secondly, it fosters and shapes a whole generation of consumers.

The Milky Way: from Milk Cartons to Vending Machines

The Quebec universal School Milk Program as I knew it was launched during Minister Jean Garon's term of office, in the mid-1970s. It was under the Ministry of Agriculture's authority before being transferred to the Ministry of Education in the 1990s. It was later abolished and merged with other policies. Today, the milk carton has disappeared from several institutions and is no longer distributed except

---

* Milk was introduced in American schools in more or less the same way as in Quebec schools. For more information, http://www.fns.usda.gov/nslp/history_11.

in underprivileged areas in the framework of the "Agir autrement" and School Milk programs. The Ministry of Education still spends $7.6 million annually to provide snacks to 60,000 students in Quebec, but the school principals now choose what the snacks will be composed of.[3]

Dairy producers nevertheless figured out a good way to keep their products in schools. In seventy-five high schools (out of nearly five hundred in the province of Quebec), there are vending machines paid for by the Quebec Federation of Milk Producers. They offer plain and chocolate milk (which constitutes 80 percent of the milk sold) for about $2 per serving. Moreover, the federation donated refrigerators containing primarily dairy products to other school cafeterias.[4]

Primary schools are no exception. Dairy producers support various outreach programs, namely, since 2009, the *School Tour*, which is part of the *Grand Défi Pierre Lavoie*. This tour of schools aims to educate students ages six to twelve by "promoting healthy life habits among young people, through physical activity and healthy eating." Last year, 25,000 chocolate milk cartons were distributed as part of this event.[5] Imagine parents' reaction if Coca-Cola were to sponsor a similar "healthy" activity. And yet, a 350-ml serving of Natrel chocolate milk contains 36 g of sugar, compared to 39 g for a standard 12-oz can of Coca-Cola.

Milk, Sugar, and Sugar

Milk at school seems normal to us; we grew up with it. But if we take a closer look, we must face the facts: we are no longer at the beginning of the last century, when we had to fatten children with whatever we had on hand. These days, although our needs and knowledge have changed, the producers' practices haven't. As we saw in Chapter 2, the role milk plays in promoting bone health has been heavily criticized; in fact, it is nearly impossible to find unbiased sources claiming that it is needed to have good bones. What we do know, however, is that milk is children's primary source of saturated fat,[6] that lactose intolerance affects more than one in five Canadians,[7] and that the milk allergy is one of the most frequent. Despite all this, we continue to give cow's milk to children as if it were an essential food.

Even worse, chocolate milk is given the green light. In the USA, 70 percent of the milk consumed in schools is flavored and USDA's milk checkoff program promotes "Chocolate Milk Has Muscle" and "Raise Your Hand for Chocolate Milk" campaigns to encourage the consumption of the substance.[8] The healthy living policy implemented in 2007 in Quebec schools eliminated soft drinks and "fake juice." But chocolate milk was there to stay even

Products Targeted at Young Consumers

All dairy processors have products targeted specifically at young people: Minigo, Tubes, and Yop for Yoplait; Crush, Coolision, and Danino for Dannon; Ficello for Parmalat, etc. Mascots, attractive colors, fun names: creativity abounds when it comes to wooing the new generation. But isn't commercial advertising aimed at children prohibited in Quebec? Yes. Except that the law doesn't cover packaging.

though it is far too sweet. According to the World Health Organization, "free sugars" (added sugars and fruit juices) should not make up more than 10 percent of the calories consumed each day. For a daily intake of two thousand calories, this corresponds to 50 g of sugar—and many nutritionists think that's still too much. One serving of the popular TruMoo strawberry milk sold in American school contains 21g of sugar[9] while a single carton of chocolate milk alone contains 30 g.[10]

The Ministry of Education recommends serving only flavored milks containing less than 30 g of sugar per cup. "This recommendation was made upon the consideration that flavored milk has good nutritional value (it contains calcium, protein, vitamins A and D)," said Esther Chouinard, spokesperson for the Ministry.[11,12] You really have to believe that cow's milk has near-miraculous properties to agree to consume a food that is such a big source of sugar when there are so many unsweetened, healthier sources of these nutrients!

But some do resist. British celebrity chef Jamie Oliver embarked on a crusade against flavored milks, an initiative that is an integral part of his "food revolution."[13] In the United States, the cafeterias of the Los Angeles Unified School District, the second-largest school district in the country, stopped offering flavored milk in the fall of 2011, following the lead of other districts. In Quebec, chocolate milk is still presented as a lesser evil to encourage children to drink milk, and it is even associated with sporting activities.

What about yogurt, then? Not much better. Consumers' magazine *Protégez-vous* analyzed the top-selling yogurts in Quebec. All children's yogurts contained between 22 and

28 g of sugar per serving.[14] A child eating one yogurt as a snack and a serving of chocolate milk with his or her lunch would already have exceeded the daily added-sugars limit recommended by the World Health Organization.

When you think about it, is it really necessary to consume so much sugar just to absorb nutrients that can easily be found elsewhere? These days, young people suffer mainly from obesity, not protein deficiency! Whereas in Quebec more than one in five children is overweight (seven percent suffer from obesity and 15 percent are overweight), we sell them sweetened milk to protect them against hypothetical diseases.[15]

Nutrition Education

It was not enough to have children drink cow's milk to stimulate consumption. Dairy producers clearly realized that they had to appeal to moms as well. "Nutrition" campaigns began during World War II. At that time, milk sales were still declining. The government had cut subsidies, which drove up prices. Meanwhile, soft drinks were gaining in popularity. As a result, producers and distributors were struggling with major surpluses.[16]

For the industry, the problem was clearly not over-production but under-consumption. Canadians did not consume the minimum amounts recommended by the *Food Guide*. Since they were unable to cut prices, the industry tried to stimulate demand through advertising. In 1948, the Association des distributeurs de lait (dairy distributors association) created an advertising agency, the "La santé par le lait" (Health through Milk) foundation. Newspaper, radio, and billboard ads appeared throughout the province, with slogans such as "Drink lots of milk," "Four glasses of milk a day no matter what," "The fluid that makes you solid," and "Drink one pint from sunrise to sunset." Although the purpose—selling more milk—is crystal clear, the foundation denied having purely mercantile goals, saying that they were doing "in-depth work to permanently instill healthy eating habits in the population."[17]

The foundation also had a large field presence. A nutritionist visited schools, parks, and homemakers' circles to distribute educational booklets, pamphlets, and films. Several messages were written by pediatricians and physicians. "Scientific data" were widely used and "experts" provided the industry with the desired legitimacy.

In a lecture given to the Association des industriels laitiers (dairy industry association) in the 1950s, nutritionist Marcelle Godbout praised the merits and superiority of educational advertising compared to commercial advertising: "In the long term, educational advertising is more profitable for the dairy industry because it seeks to permanently change eating habits, and thus promotes a substantial increase in cow's milk consumption."[18] Ms. Godbout went on to note that "only recognized experts with degrees are able to perform the scientific popularization work related to educational advertising."[19]

Even today, Dairy Farmers of Canada is investing millions of dollars each year in nutrition research and has established partnerships with the leading Canadian universities. DFC employs about twenty dietitians who work hard to produce informational materials aimed at each province and each audience. For DFC, nutrition is purely and simply marketing: every opportunity to praise the merits of milk and show it in a good light must be taken.

Got Advertising?

But providing health arguments is clearly not enough: our food choices are also a matter of emotion, and the Quebec Federation of Milk Producers has realized this. There is no denying that the promotional campaigns produced over the past thirty years have played an important role in our commitment to cow's milk. It all started with an observation made in the early 1980s. At that time, soft drinks were becoming increasingly popular, while milk sales were declining again. Young people who had been heavy consumers of milk in their childhood now felt embarrassed to drink it in public. Milk was for babies. The demand, therefore, had to be stimulated by changing the product's image from a symbol of parental authority to an instrument of self-affirmation that is cool and desirable in society, just like coffee, soft drinks, or beer.[20]

That's when Normand Brathwaite came onto the scene. Still little known at the time, the young actor had been discovered mainly for his performances in the Ligue nationale d'improvisation. In 1984, he was hired to promote milk, a choice that reflected the significant sociological changes happening in Quebec society, which was becoming increasingly ethnically diverse. It was a risky but winning bet: Normand Brathwaite quickly became a star and embodied the idea that consuming milk was a way to assert oneself, to stand out from the others, and to be healthy. In every ad, he is surrounded by beautiful young smiling people who affirm to the world that they are great and drink what's best: milk. At the front of my third-grade class, we had a poster of him, smiling a big toothy grin, a glass of milk in his hand. It was signed with the slogan: "Milk, frankly the best."

Roch Voisine and Nostalgia

But the school market was not enough. In an article published in the history journal *Cap-aux-diamants*, Nicole Dubé, marketing director of the Quebec Federation of Milk Producers, explains how, after children, the over-thirty group became the industry's new target: "Our strategy is twofold: a rational approach and an emotional approach. The former presents milk as a significant source of calcium and a first-choice weapon in the fight against osteoporosis, while the latter showcases the joyful reunion of consumers and milk."[21]

After several years of campaigning with Normand Brathwaite as a spokesperson, milk consumption among adults was still insufficient in Nicole Dubé's view. She decided to stigmatize "adults who are full of praise for cow's milk, while drinking little or none at all."[22] They must be made to face their own hypocrisy! The Federation found the perfect person to address Quebecers in Roch Voisine: "His role as an actor promoting milk had Roch speaking openly to men about their contradictory behavior; he also knew how to reach women by reminding them of our desire to see our loved ones make the best choices for their health."

In the late 1990s, producers abandoned popular spokesmen and turned to nostalgia. Because nostalgia is an emotion that sells. Using music by Gilbert Bécaud, Joe

Dassin, and Dalida, the dairy producers associated milk with good memories. The advertising images used white as a primary color and were carefully polished and composed, focusing on childhood, a first love, nighttime cravings, a mother breastfeeding her baby. The "white" campaign won over the whole province. The campaign's albums on CD (*L'album blanc*, volumes I and II), a compilation of the songs used in the commercials, sold more than 280,000 copies. A portion of the profits were given to the Fondation OLO, which provides milk, eggs, and oranges to disadvantaged pregnant women.[23]

The world has changed quite a bit since the time when half-pints were sold for three cents. Yet we are told pretty much the same thing today: schoolchildren need milk because it is essential. We now know this is wrong. Our nutrition knowledge—which we acquired from sources other than our yellow activity book—convinced us to take nachos, cheeseburgers, and pizza off our plates. This same knowledge should also eject chocolate milk–vending machines from school cafeterias.

Now that we know that cow's milk is not the best source of calcium, we can see why habits, emotions, and polished images are needed to convince us to keep drinking it. And to justify the way we treat dairy cows.

6

IF COWS WERE UNHAPPY, THEY WOULDN'T PRODUCE MILK

Cows are capable of suffering, both physically and psychologically. They are social animals with complex intelligence, and they do not produce milk to make us happy. They do it because they are forced to—we artificially inseminate them, and then take their calves away from them at birth. They spend their lives tied up in stalls, without access to the outdoors, and are later sold to become ground beef.

A VIDEO OF THE AMAGEZA Rally in South Africa became popular on YouTube soon after it was uploaded. Filmed using a camera attached to the helmet of Johan Gray, one of the participants, the sequence is quite remarkable—you truly feel as if you were the one riding the motorcycle. We're with Gray on a deserted road in the middle of this fourteen-day endurance race, when we see a young calf stuck in a concrete canal filled with water. Gray makes a U-turn and stops. What will he do? This is where you can't help but be impressed by Gray's ingenuity: he ties a strap to his motorcycle and goes down into the canal. He is soon knee-deep in water. He slowly approaches the animal and gently grabs hold of it.

The challenge is now to get back on the road. After a few unsuccessful attempts, he makes it. But Gray's troubles are not over yet. What do you do with a calf in the middle of such an isolated place? He sets the calf on the seat of his BMW, as if it were the most natural thing in the world, and slowly drives around in search of the owner. The farmer is soon found. A few words are exchanged, and the farmer says that the calf's mother has been calling for it tirelessly for several hours. Gray returns the animal, which rejoins its herd.

The comments on YouTube overwhelmingly applaud Gray's actions—he is a motorcyclist with heart and courage, a man willing to lose a race to help an animal in distress,

What Is Animal Ethics?

Animal ethics is the branch of ethics that deals with our obligations to animals. Generally, the existence of animal suffering is key. Indeed, to many theorists, the relevant criterion for moral consideration should not be some human-specific intellectual faculties or the fact that an animal is alive, but rather the ability to suffer. Today, no one doubts that vertebrates (mammals, birds, and fish) are conscious and can feel pain. And if animals are sentient beings, their suffering must be taken into account. This also means that we cannot consider them as mere objects or resources to serve our purposes.

a model to emulate! But wait just a minute. Johan Gray doesn't seem to be a vegan. He eats meat and cheese. The life he bravely saved belongs to an animal who will provide milk for his cereal or become his dinner a few months from now. Why are we willing to make great sacrifices to save one animal while we exploit thousands of others and think nothing of it? Maybe because we don't really know what a cow's life is like. Perhaps because it seems easier to take action when faced with a given individual whom we can clearly identify—a calf in a canal—rather than anonymous masses. Perhaps, finally, because we find it convenient to think it's okay to eat and exploit animals.

A Cow's Life

The sky is so blue and the grass so green on milk cartons! How could cows not feel free and happy in such a bucolic setting? I have seen many Quebec landscapes that make you want to roll in the grass, but there were never any cows grazing freely in them. And for good reason—that's not where they live. They do not spend their days lounging in pastures, grazing on clover. Just take a walk through the Warwick area to the south-east of Montreal and you will see that, apart from a few heifers (future dairy cows), there are no cows in the pastures. In fact, there are no pastures either, only soybean fields as far as the eye can see. So, where have the cows gone? They're crammed inside barns.

In Quebec, about 92 percent of the 382,000 dairy cows are housed in barns and tied in stalls so narrow that they can't turn around. The official term is "tie stalls." And it is said to be normal, or even necessary. "Using tie stalls enables us to produce more milk by providing more care to the animals—especially with regard to nutrition and reproduction," says Robert Séguin, a Sainte-Marthe dairy producer.[1] A necessary evil then? In Ontario, the percentage of cows living in stalls is much lower (71.9 percent) and in the rest of Canada, the majority are free. In the U.S., almost three out of every four lactating cows are housed in freestall or dry lot areas.[2]* Elsewhere in the world, in the Netherlands, for example, only 10 percent of cows are tied in their stalls.[3]

In addition to being often tied up, dairy cows almost never go outside. In the view of François Dumontier, spokesperson for the Quebec Federation of Milk Producers, "beyond the bucolic factor, it's not so clear that going outside is an advantage for the cow."[4] Nonetheless, if given a choice, cows do prefer to go outside when weather permits, as a research team from the University of British Columbia discovered in 2010 after conducting a study in which a group of twenty-five cows was given complete freedom of movement. The cows spent 46 percent of their day indoors, especially in hot weather. On the other hand, they preferred to spend their night outside. For a cow, the best of all worlds is thus a barn with open doors.[5] However, farmland prices are such that the decision to use land to grow crops instead of grazing cows is understandable.

Dairy cows also spend their entire lives bearing calves. A cow's life is in fact essentially a series of inseminations

---

* Cows in freestall barns are not restrained and are free to enter, lie down, stand up, and leave the barn whenever they desire. A dry lot is an open lot that has no vegetative cover used as primary cow housing in the more arid climate.

and calvings. We tend to forget that cows do not naturally produce milk all year round. Like women, they produce milk only after giving birth. Except that as soon as cows have calved, we inseminate them and they become pregnant again. On average, they lactate seven out of the nine months of their pregnancy, which leaves them very little time to rest.

Cows are not "designed" to produce milk like that. They do not give milk because they are happy. They do it because we force them to and because they've been genetically selected based on their ability to produce. And it works—today, our cows produce twice as much milk as they did in the 1960s.[6]

Performance Machines

Milk production is by no means a craft. It's more clever engineering to improve performance. Data and quantitative analysis are the lifeblood of this industry. As a cow is worth thousands of dollars and will produce for only three or four years, it is essential to achieve optimal genetics to ensure the best yields.[7]

While a cow "naturally" produces seven kg of milk per day, under current conditions, an animal yields 27 kg per day. With this significant increase in productivity comes an enormous physical demand. John Webster, professor emeritus at the Bristol Veterinary School of Medicine in the United Kingdom and specialist in animal welfare issues, puts the daily effort now required from a cow "on a par with jogging six or more hours a day or competing in the Tour de France."[8] It comes as no surprise that this high level of milk production is detrimental to the welfare of cows, as Dr. Olivier Berreville, biologist and scientific advisor for Canadians for the Ethical Treatment of Farm Animals (CETFA) explains: "Cows often develop metabolic disorders and infections such as mastitis, a painful inflammation of the udder. The large volume of their udders may also force the animals to walk with their hind legs wide apart, which causes lameness."[9] The use of rBST (see Chapter 3) exacerbates the health problems that already plague dairy cows. According to the *Canadian Journal of Veterinary Research*, "Cows treated with rBST face a nearly 25% increase in the risk of clinical mastitis, a 40% reduction in fertility, and a 55% increase in the risk of lameness."[10]

Producing this much milk requires such a significant amount of energy that grazing in a meadow wouldn't be enough to meet the cow's needs. Her naturally herbivorous diet is thus replaced by a specific mixture of fodder and grains fortified with vitamins and minerals. To maximize the energy intake, cows are fed a diet rich in grains and low in fiber, which causes them digestive problems. Acidosis, an imbalance of the rumen pH, is one of the most common diseases and unfortunately one that is hard to diagnose. It causes diarrhea and can be fatal.[11]

Finally, again with the aim of optimizing performance, cows are mutilated. Heifer calves are regularly dehorned (or their horn buds are ablated) without anesthetic. A cow's tail may also be amputated without any painkillers being administered. This practice is also quite pointless: contrary to popular belief, docking a cow's tail doesn't help keep the udder and legs any cleaner, nor does it reduce the risk of mammary infection.[12] It is also not uncommon for females to be born with one or more additional teats, and these are often cut off by the dairy farmers so that the udder is better suited to the number of teat cups on the milking machines.

Crying like a Baby
Cows' suffering is not only physical. It is also—mostly—emotional. Each year, a cow gives birth to a baby who is systematically taken away from her at birth. In nature, calves suckle for six to nine months and are weaned gradually; heifer calves usually stay with their mothers for life and bull calves for one year, after which they leave the herd. On modern farms, newborn calves are immediately isolated in individual boxes or stalls, depriving them of physical contact and social interaction. This separation is necessary, since the cow must produce milk for the milking machine, not for her young. But this parting creates a terrible feeling of

Starbuck, the Alpha Male

Starbuck was the name given to a bull who was born in Hanoverhill, Ontario, on April 26, 1979, and died in Saint-Hyacinthe nineteen years later. Starbuck is undoubtedly the most virile male in Canadian history. His exceptional genetics made him an insemination star. In total, more than 685,000 vials of his seed were sold in forty-five countries for revenues of nearly $25 million.[13] This means that all Canadian Holstein cows may be able to trace their family tree back to Starbuck.

anguish on both sides. As Dr. Berreville sees it, this practice is a very traumatic experience for the animals: "Isolation can cause both psychological and physiological stress in calves and compromise their immune system, which can lead to illnesses and even death. The separation is also a significant source of distress for mothers, who may call to their calves for several days after the event." Professor John Webster has described the removal of the calf as the "most potentially distressing incident in the life of the dairy cow."[14] He also noted that "the cow will submit herself to considerable personal discomfort or risk to nourish and protect her calf."

American veterinarian Holly Cheever experienced this first hand. One anecdote she related left me profoundly upset.[15] It happened near Syracuse, New York, in the early 1980s. At that time, many cows still had access to the outside, which is not the case today. A cow gave birth alone in a field. As usual, she brought her calf to the barn shortly after. The mother was in good shape and, between the morning and evening milkings, she was free to graze in a large pasture. But the owner was worried. The cow's udder was empty— she produced virtually no milk. After several days with no sign of milk coming in, he called upon Dr. Cheever, who examined the animal and found nothing wrong. The farmer continued to investigate. It was not until a little later that he found the explanation to this problem by following his cow to the far end of the pasture. She went there to join another calf. It turned out that eleven days earlier, she had given birth to twins and no one had realized there was a second calf. After four calvings and all of her little ones being ripped away, it was the first time she was finally able to nurse one of her offspring. Despite Dr. Cheever's pleas, the calf emptying its mother's udder was taken away. That cow in Syracuse was not to be distracted from her real purpose: to produce milk. For humans.

Dr. Cheever doesn't say what happened to the calf the cow had kept hidden. But it's quite easy to guess. Like the others, the animal was bottle-fed with a powdered milk preparation. If she was a heifer, she became a dairy cow in her turn. If he was a bull, since he didn't have the genetic characteristics to be raised as beef cattle, he was sold at auction for a few dollars. He would then have been fattened for twenty weeks or so before being sent to the slaughterhouse to become veal.

Dumb as a Cow?

The sad story of the cow who wanted to take care of her calf reminds us that despite the prejudices humans harbor against them, cattle are capable of complex reasoning. This cow first had to remember her previous babies that she had never seen again. She then probably devised and executed some kind of plan: if leaving her young babies to the breeder meant losing them, then she would have to hide them. Finally, rather than concealing both calves, which would have aroused the farmer's suspicions, she let him take one of the two.

Does Dr. Cheever think that the cow in Syracuse was really able to design and carry out a plan like that? She prefers not to speculate, but cannot help feeling empathy for the animal: "I cannot tell you how she knew to do this—it would seem more likely that a desperate mother would hide both. All I know is this: there is a lot more going on behind those beautiful eyes than we humans have ever given them credit for, and as a mother who was able to nurse all four of my babies and did not have to suffer the agonies of losing my beloved offspring, I feel her pain."[16]

Cows don't show affection only to their calves—they also have complex social structures and are extremely attached to one another. John Webster documented how they form small groups of friends within a herd. Most often, they meet in groups of two, three, or four, and spend most of their time grooming and licking each other. They may also dislike other cows and hold grudges against them for months or years.[17] It is not known whether they gossip about each other or if they comment on the farmer's clothes, but otherwise they have just about everything it takes to be a real group of girlfriends. They also develop relationships with the human beings around them. In *The Secret Life of Cows*, Rosamund Young describes how cows who anticipate a difficult birth or are worried about the well-being of other cows will seek assistance from humans.[18]

Pleasure in Problem Solving

Professor Donald Broom of Cambridge University studies the behavior of cows. His team created a special pen in which they installed a lever that, when pressed, grants access to a field full of all kinds of foods that cows love. In short, pushing the lever takes you to a small (cattle) paradise. When the cows figured out how to operate it, they showed unmistakable signs of joy: "Their heart rates increased and they were more likely to jump and gallop when they went down towards the food. It was as if the animals were saying 'Eureka! I've found out how to solve the problem.'"[19]

Findings such as these do not necessarily require a complicated device. An Irish farmer was recently able to see first-hand how clever cows are. He found it strange that every night, the stable door opened and his animals took to the open fields. To get to the bottom of it, he left a camera recording in the building all night. The next morning, the mystery was solved. One of the cows, Daisy, had learned how to open the two latches on the door with her tongue to let her friends out. The story was covered in a television report in which the journalist described Daisy as a "Bovine Einstein."[20]

Auctions: A Purgatory that Does Not Lead to Paradise
Before ending their lives at the slaughterhouse, cows must go through one last crucial step: auctions. They are brought to one of Quebec's six auctions to be sold to wholesalers. These auctions are public and I visited the one in Saint-Isidore, Beauce.

The auction takes place in a huge modern building with a welcoming lobby where receptionists work busily behind a glass wall. "A 2,000-head capacity," says the website. Without the traces of dirt on the floor and the persistent barn odor, you could imagine you were standing in a medical clinic. Upstairs, there is a huge cafeteria with a stadium-type menu: fries, burgers, corndogs, and so on. A dozen men in their fifties and sixties are rushing to finish their plates. An announcement over the intercom has just informed them that the auctions are about to begin. They get up, leaving their trays on the table. I follow them.

The whole group goes into a large room where concrete bleachers overlook something that resembles a stage with a dirt floor. People sit down. I take a seat behind them. The auctioneer and his assistant are standing behind a large wall with a small window in it. On our left, metal doors open. A young man confidently sporting a mullet pushes the first cow forward with a whip. She walks a few steps and then he hits her to make her turn around. Her weight—1,200 pounds—is displayed on a screen. I learn that auction sales start at $0.60 a pound and that's pretty much all I can grasp from the auctioneer's uninterrupted flow of words.

I cannot help but remember the price of ground beef at the grocery store: about $4 a pound. The margins are low. Every cent counts. I see calculators appear, some people taking notes, hands being raised discreetly. Sold! The young man with the whip pushes the cow that has just been sold through the right-hand exit just as another one takes her place. And another. And another. And another. As each new cow is brought in, the sound of the metal doors makes me jump. I find myself unable to look at the animals, so I try to focus on the person bringing them in and taking them out. Whose task it is to make them move so that people can see how plump and fit they are.

The atmosphere is tense. Large sums of money are exchanged. Each cow sells for between $700 and $1,000. An animal that is too weak and doesn't survive transportation is a net loss. Intermediaries who will sell the cows to the slaughterhouse must also ensure that they get a good price once the animals arrive.

An Unhappy Ending

Regardless of their sensitivity and intelligence, dairy cows, who can live up to twenty years, are usually slaughtered after four years, once their productivity begins to decrease. Their flesh becomes ground beef. Burgers from the major chains in Quebec are, therefore, made of recycled dairy cows.

In the province of Quebec, 70,000 "cull cows" (cows who are retired after four years) are produced annually; until recently, they were all sent to the Levinoff-Colbex slaughterhouse in St-Cyrille-de-Wendover near Drummondville. However, the facility, which is owned by the Quebec Federation of Cattle Producers, was forced to suspend its activities in spring 2012 due to major financial difficulties. It was the last major slaughterhouse specializing in cull cows in eastern Canada. Pierre-Paul Noreau, editorial writer for *Le Soleil*, claims that it was not necessary to have this type of facility in Quebec: "The Quebec market for cull animals is simply too small and external competition too fierce, especially with regard to the U.S. market, given the current strength of the Canadian dollar."[21]

Much has been said about the economic issues regarding the closure of the Levinoff-Colbex slaughterhouse, but this decision also has a significant impact on the retired cows. The suspension of the facility's operations means that the animals from Quebec must be transported over 700 more kilometers. They are sold at auctions where intermediaries acquire them and then transport them to slaughterhouses located in Guelph, Ontario, or Pennsylvania.[22]

Behind me, at the top of the bleachers, large doors lead to a footbridge that allows you to walk above the cows. To my right, a few hundred cows are waiting for their turn to be sold. To my left, the ones that have just been purchased are crammed ten to an enclosure. The udders of some cows are so big that they seem about to burst. The joints of some of the others are swollen. I see a group of cows lying on the ground, breathing with difficulty. One man, his cap molded tightly to his head, approaches me: "Those ones are going to have a hard time getting to Guelph." I ask him what they'll do with these cows. "We'll put fewer in the truck, to give them a chance." He describes his job to me enthusiastically. He buys cull cows from milk producers, loads them on his truck, and sells them here. His have just been sold. He got a good price. He has a light heart and feels like chatting.

I explore further. I open a new door and find myself in another auction room identical to the first. Except that here they sell calves who are just a few days old. It's simply impossible not to fall for these animals struggling to stand on their feet. I take a seat. The auctioneer (the brother of the other one, someone has told me) looks at me and smiles: "Would you like a little calf, madam?" I ask him how much they cost. "Thirty bucks." Cheaper than a cat. The image of a calf grazing in my yard pops into my mind. I see him grow, but I also imagine the looks on my neighbors' faces. I shake my head. The calf is sold. He will go to a "finisher" and be slaughtered in about twenty weeks' time.

Dr. Berreville has attended many auctions, and what I saw was nothing special. As he explained, "The auction environment is not favorable to the welfare of animals. Some cows arrive there emaciated, suffering from infections and diseases caused by milk overproduction, and are often treated brutally. They are in transit for an average of three weeks between the farm and the slaughterhouse, going from auction to auction until the producers get what they deem to be a fair price. Because of all this, it's not uncommon for animals to become non-ambulatory [unable to stand or move without help]. Yet, even those who suffer severely are generally not euthanized. CETFA inspectors and I have documented—with photos and video footage—many cases of suffering animals that were being dragged behind the buildings of the auction and left there, dying, without care."

It is relatively easy to visit stables and auctions, but the doors of slaughterhouses remain closed to visitors. Only those who work there can see, hear, and sense the death of the animals. To write his doctoral thesis, which later became the book *Every Twelve Seconds: Industrialized Slaughter and the Politics of Sight*,[23] American political scientist Timothy Pachirat got a job as a slaughterhouse worker. For five months, day after day, he noted his observations on the power relationships and the challenges killing all day long present to workers. In reading his testimony, we come to see how torture and suffering in slaughterhouses are not accidental. They're just part of the routine—the volume of kills is such that it is simply impossible to treat the animals decently. The animals, who form a continuous flow (one killing every twelve seconds, hence the title of the book), are not considered individuals but rather raw materials. Cattle are called "meat" while they are still alive, which helps employees avoid realizing the full extent of what they are doing.

We must face facts: there is no moral distinction between milk and meat. The same animals are milked, then sold and finally slaughtered. Calves, cows, steers, they are all auctioned and slaughtered sooner or later! And if one really wants to differentiate their situations, then a cow's fate is probably less enviable than a steer's, since steers have a much shorter life and enjoy a little more freedom.

Let's be clear. Our current system hides the fact that cows are sentient beings capable of emotions, mammals with a nervous system similar to ours. We treat them as mere milk-producing machines. Simply because we find it convenient. American legal scholar Gary L. Francione, who advocates the abolition of all animal exploitation, sums up the situation perfectly: "There is probably more suffering in a glass of milk or an ice cream cone than there is in a steak."[24]

Are We Carnists?

We eat eggs and animals and drink milk without a second thought. This is what we've always done and it seems normal. This practice is based on a system of implicit beliefs that psychologist Melanie Joy calls "carnism." Carnism is the ideology (a structured set of values and beliefs) according to

The Veal Roast, a By-Product of the Dairy Industry

What happens to male calves after they're purchased at the auction? There are two main ways to "finish" (fatten) them: they can be "milk fed" or "grain fed." Grain-fed calves are given enriched corn until their slaughter at the age of six months. Milk-fed calves, on the other hand, are confined in individual wooden stalls and given powdered milk. People often think that their flesh is whiter because of the milk they drink, but it is actually because they are deprived of iron. In Europe, rearing calves in cubicles is prohibited.

which it is morally acceptable to eat certain animals. This ideology is obviously in opposition to veganism.

In her book *Why We Love Dogs, Eat Pigs, and Wear Cows: An Introduction to Carnism*,[25] Joy explains how, in our societies, consuming meat, eggs, and dairy products is considered a fact of life rather than an option. Yet, it is an actual choice, since we do not need to eat animal-based foods to survive. Our ancestors may very well have had to, but today a typical North American or European can be perfectly healthy—and enjoy plenty of opportunities to satisfy his or her taste buds—while being strictly vegan. Indeed, the official position of the American Dietetic Association and Dietitians of Canada is clear: "[A]ppropriately planned vegetarian diets are healthy, nutritionally adequate, and provide health benefits in the prevention and treatment of certain diseases."[26,27] Like it or not, consuming meat or milk is a matter of moral choice.

If I Look at the Mass, I Will Never Act

Why would someone take the risk of stopping on the side of the road, going down in a canal, damaging his clothes, and losing precious minutes in a timed competition to save a single calf while millions of cows lead the life that I have just described above, and nobody's doing anything for them?

This problem is the same one that American psychologist Paul Slovic discusses in an article titled "If I Look at the Mass, I Will Never Act."[28] The title is originally a quote from Mother Teresa. In his text, Slovic tries to understand our lack of action when faced with large numbers. While we are caring people who would make an enormous effort to rescue a victim in front of us, we become indifferent to the misery of the same individuals who, in a broader context, are seen merely as "one among many others." Slovic thus analyzes the fundamental mechanisms that lead us to ignore human disasters.

I think that the same mechanisms can explain why we are in general only marginally affected by the conditions in which animals are reared or slaughtered. We need to feel emotions before we will act. Statistics on the number of fatalities or casualties, however, fail to communicate the real meaning of the atrocities. We know that these events are real, but we do not feel their reality. These are just numbers, and numbers are not enough to elicit the emotional responses that motivate action.

This is where the carnist ideology comes into play, suggesting that the problem does not even exist because eating meat and drinking milk are "normal" behaviors. As with sexism or racism, carnism is based on the idea that "this is how things are." In many cultures, it is "normal" for women to be treated as inferior to men. It is also "normal" for some people to be treated differently because they don't have the same skin color as the others. Similarly, it is "normal" to consume and exploit some animals.

In all these cases, the "norm" conceals an ideology (sexism, racism, and carnism) that seeks to make us accept values as mere facts. Yet we are perfectly free to choose to combat these ideologies if we believe in a few principles, like welfare, justice, autonomy, or compassion. I think it's even a moral duty.

Avoiding that Guilty Feeling

Even when we know the reasons for taking action, and even

when we want to be just and compassionate people, it seems difficult to make the leap and change our behavior toward animals—starting with our diet. Why aren't we more ethical?

I posed this question to Dr. Martin Gibert, philosopher and author of *Voir son steak comme un animal mort* (loosely translated, the title means "looking at your steak and seeing a dead animal"), a book about moral psychology and veganism.[29] He explained that we often lack the willpower or rationality. For example, we may have very good reasons to quit smoking, but this doesn't mean it will be easy to stop. In this case, it is more of a willingness issue. But we also tend to bend our reasoning so that it aligns with our intuitions. We look for *post hoc* justifications when our decisions are already made.

Still, consuming animals remains difficult, psychologically speaking. "Many people vaguely realize they should not be eating meat," says Gibert. "At the same time, they really like it. And social norms say it's okay to eat meat. This is changing slowly, but socially, it's still the norm. In moral psychology, this is called the 'paradox of meat.' It means we must deal with a particular form of cognitive dissonance: on the one hand, our love for animals, our denial of cruelty, our disgust for slaughterhouses, and on the other hand, our taste for meat. We have developed a strategy to mitigate this paradox, attributing lower levels of consciousness to the animals we eat. It's a way of telling ourselves, 'These animals that I eat, they're not really conscious, they don't really suffer.'"[30]

There are other strategies too. Gibert has identified one that applies perfectly to dairy products. The idea is for us to use the possibility of appropriate treatment of animals—a potential world free from suffering—as justification for not changing our practices in the real world. The argument is a weak one, but it satisfies our reasoning.* Moreover, it is not inaccurate to say that, in theory, we could have cruelty-free animal products. This idea is addressed in the book *Zoopolis* by Will Kymlicka and Sue Donaldson,[31] who discuss a hypothetical vegan utopia where animals would somehow be fellow citizens endowed with fundamental rights. In short, a human/animal relationship devoid of abuse or domination—an ideal world from a moral perspective. Donaldson and Kymlicka argue that, in this context, we could not eat animals, but consuming eggs and milk might be acceptable. It would certainly prove uneconomical, as we'd have to content ourselves with the surplus milk that remains when the calf has finished suckling and doesn't want more. But it is indeed possible for us to imagine cruelty-free milk.

For Gibert, it is precisely this kind of theoretical possibility that the human mind uses to alleviate certain cognitive dissonances: "When we're about to consume milk, even if we know it has been produced under unacceptable conditions, we can still tell ourselves that it could have been produced without any suffering. This is obviously a very bad argument. But I think that this mere possibility is enough for us to stop feeling guilty. And I think it works very well with dairy products because they are not directly related to the flesh—they don't directly involve death."

To sum up, we are very good at justifying our consumption of milk by keeping the suffering of cows out of the picture,

---

* More technically, Gibert suggests calling this type of faulty reasoning "upward counterfactual bias."

by letting ourselves believe that they're happy to produce milk. Unfortunately, we can't rely solely on our intuitions to act appropriately. Because as we know, they may very well be sexist, racist, or carnist.

We must therefore use our reason too (a separate faculty from intuition) to answer questions like "What should I do?," "What should I eat?," or "What should I drink?" However, from a rational point of view, if we believe that no sentient being should be mistreated or exploited, then opting for a vegan diet—without any animal products—appears to be the most consistent moral attitude. If we have the choice (and most of us do), I don't see how we can justify causing animals to suffer just for our pleasure.

It may very well be impossible to go completely vegan, just as it's probably impossible to never tell a lie and always be a good person. Each context is different and comes with its own share of constraints. The idea is not to reach purity and perfection, but to recognize that in most cases, the best thing to do is to avoid exploiting animals, and to move toward this moral rule.

Maybe you don't come to the same conclusions that I do. Maybe you think we can solve everything with the adoption of laws that protect animals, or that we can get around the problem by opting for milk produced on organic farms. In the next two chapters, we will see that the governments currently don't protect livestock in any way and that premium-priced organic milk, very unfortunately, isn't produced without suffering.

7

ANIMAL ABUSE IS ILLEGAL

When it comes to legislation, everything is set up to make it seem that cows and other farm animals are treated well. Unfortunately, this remains largely theoretical. In reality, dairy cows do not really have any legal protection, and the industry is allowed to decide what is to be considered acceptable practice

IN SPRING 2012, NATIONAL ASSEMBLY of Quebec member and opposition agriculture critic, André Simard, made headlines when he spoke out against ritual slaughter. People of the Muslim faith generally follow halal standards, according to which an animal must be blessed by an Imam before being put to death by having its throat slit while it is still conscious. In the view of Simard, a veterinarian by training, this practice "may cause unnecessary suffering to the animal."[1] His words earned him much criticism, some people even labeling him a racist. He was quick to correct these views, explaining, "It's not a religious debate. It's a debate about standards." Simard wants the spirit of the law to be respected, which is to say that the animal ought to be unconscious at the time of slaughter.

We should all welcome the fact that an elected official is trying to prevent the unnecessary suffering of animals. The problem is that animals don't suddenly become aware and sentient only fifteen minutes before their slaughter. Throughout their lives, they are treated like machines and are largely unprotected by the law. If we are moved by their suffering, it is not slaughter standards that we should address as a priority, but the whole body of legislation governing the lives of animals. There is an urgent need for action: year after year, Quebec consistently takes the prize for Canada's worst province in terms of animal welfare.[2]

An Exception that Disproves the Rule

Yet laws do exist. The Animal Health Protection Act (R.S.Q. c. P-42) currently in force in Quebec clearly states that all animals must be treated well. The problem comes from the exceptions embedded in that law.

The Act reads as follows: "The owner or custodian of an animal shall ensure that the safety and welfare of the animal are not jeopardized. The safety or welfare of an animal is jeopardized where:

1. the animal does not have access to drinking water or food in quantities and of a quality in keeping with its biological requirements;

2. the animal is not kept in premises that are suitable, salubrious, clean and adapted to the animal's biological requirements and where the installations are not likely to affect the animal's safety or welfare or is not properly transported in an appropriate vehicle;

3. the animal does not receive the health care required by its condition while it is wounded, sick or suffering;
4. the animal is subject to abuse or ill-treatment that may affect its health."[3]

In other words, when we are the owner or custodian of an animal, we must provide it with adequate care. The law was actually amended to include protection for all domestic animals—which technically includes farm animals. Until that change was made, this section covered only cats and dogs. So what is the loophole? As soon as an animal is being used in the framework of an agricultural activity, it is excluded from protection altogether. No matter what the agricultural activity is, provided that this activity is practiced "in accordance with generally accepted rules"—which is to say, the common industry practices—it is exempt from the section of the law covering animal welfare. This basically means, "You have rights, but those rights stop at the doors of the barn."

Are there other laws that could protect dairy cows? I asked Sophie Gaillard, lawyer and campaigns manager for the Montreal SPCA's Animal Advocacy Department.

Gaillard explained that, in theory, animals could fall under the protection of the Canadian Criminal Code that contains provisions dealing with animal cruelty. And in the Criminal Code there is no exemption for agricultural activities. But in practice, things are more complicated: "The problem," she said, "is that the way the main section of this part of the Code has been formulated and the way this section has been interpreted by courts in the past makes applying the

Criminal Code to the agricultural context very difficult. The Code makes it illegal to intentionally cause unnecessary pain, suffering, or injury. One would therefore have to be able to prove that the pain, suffering, or injury inflicted on the dairy cow was not necessary. Though old and therefore potentially outdated, case law on this issue suggests that when the practice in question is part of the food industry's standard operations, it is not unnecessary. . . . We have to eat after all!"[4]

The Criminal Code and case law thus create some form of de facto exemption for animals used in agriculture, just as provincial law does more explicitly. As long as the treatments and practices to which dairy cows are subjected are "normal" in the industry, they appear to be legitimate. Bad news for our cows.

Existing legislation allows producers to decide for themselves what is "appropriate" or not in terms of animal well-being. Only purely malicious and gratuitous torture caused without any intention to increase the animal's productivity, and condemned by the industry itself, appears to be a punishable offence. There are also national codes of practice establishing minimum livestock welfare standards (the one pertaining to dairy cows is currently being reviewed), but for the time being, compliance with these codes is strictly on a voluntary basis in the vast majority of provinces.

Live Fast . . . Die Young

Dairy cows are not protected by any legislation during their productive lives, and the end of their existence follows the same lines. Their transportation and slaughter are effectively covered by certain federal and provincial legislation (which slaughter following certain religious rites would violate), but the regulations promulgated under these laws have a number of loopholes.

Some provisions have the advantage of being clear: animals of different species, for example, must be segregated during transport and the pens in which they wait to be slaughtered must be fitted with water troughs (if they are to be kept there more than a certain number of hours). However, many articles refer to subjective concepts that are relatively difficult to assess. For example, the federal meat inspection regulations, which apply to federally inspected slaughterhouses, state that, "No food animal shall be handled in a manner that subjects the animal to avoidable distress or avoidable pain." But what constitutes "avoidable distress or avoidable pain"? Furthermore, the agency responsible for enforcing these laws and regulations, the Canadian Food Inspection Agency (CFIA), is described in the latest report from the World Society for the Protection of Animals[5] as

Are American Dairy Cows Any Luckier?

Much like in Quebec, animals used for food production in the U.S. are afforded virtually no legal protection, whether at the federal or state level. The Animal Welfare Act, which constitutes the primary piece of federal animal protection legislation in the U.S., completely exempts farm animals. The federal Humane Slaughter Act, which requires that slaughter "be carried out only by humane methods" to prevent "needless suffering" excludes poultry from its application, meaning that over 95 percent of all animals killed for food are not protected from inhumane slaughter. Finally, the Twenty-Eight-Hour Law, a federal law that governs the transport of farm animals, has been interpreted by the U.S. Department of Agriculture as only applicable to transport by a railcar, despite the fact that the vast majority of American livestock is transported by truck.

At the state level, the only available protection for farm animals lies in criminal anti-cruelty legislation. State anti-cruelty laws generally take one of two forms. First, some statutes adopt similar language to the Canadian Criminal Code: they prohibit "unjustifiable" or "unnecessary" suffering to animals, leaving courts free to interpret these vague and subjective terms to mean that standard industrial farming practices are not legally cruel because they are "necessary" for the purposes of food production, even if they cause a tremendous degree of suffering. However, most states use the same formula as Quebec's Animal Health Protection Act and simply exempt all "accepted," "common," "customary," or "normal" agricultural practices, effectively denying any legal protection to farm animals. Thus, as a practical matter, American dairy cows are not by any means better protected than their Quebec counterparts.[6]

particularly lax about the ways animals are treated. In short, the law is rife with loopholes and there is no one to enforce it.

We Can Do Better

Many people believe that with more restrictive laws, producers could not stay in business. Sophie Gaillard responds by citing the example of Switzerland, a country where the dairy industry is highly regulated: "There, the law dictates the conditions in which cows are to be raised in great detail (covering, for example, lighting, space, ground, food, etc.), tail docking is prohibited, and dairy cows that are kept tethered must be allowed to go outdoors on a regular basis, at least ninety days per year, and must not spend more than two weeks without access to outdoors."

The situation for cows in Quebec is still a long way from that. Gaillard maintains that we should at least establish standards of care governing the treatment of cows during their time on the farm. "The fact that no law protects them during this period (which corresponds to most of their productive life) and that the industry is left completely to itself is outrageous," she says. "Would we trust the oil industry to determine what constitutes an acceptable level of pollution?"

A Code of Good Intentions

In 2009, Dairy Farmers of Canada published the "Code of Practice for the Care and Handling of Dairy Cattle."[7] It contains some general requirements, such as "Build stalls to minimize hock and knee injuries and to allow cows to rise and lie down with ease," and "Daily removal of cow patties and use of generous amounts of bedding assures cleanliness of cows kept in bedded-pack pens." What mechanisms are in place to ensure that producers comply with the code? Are there incentives for doing so? Thérèse Beaulieu, spokesperson for the DFC, replied honestly. "We promoted the Code on several occasions, in meetings with producers and representatives of trade journals. We also tried to reach out to veterinarians as allies. [. . .] Since the Code is based on scientific research, we have data proving to producers that certain practices are profitable for them—cows live longer, being comfortable allows them to lie down for longer periods, which facilitates digestion and thus milk production. Paying attention to the cow's health is quite obviously good for milk quality."[8]

With the exception of the province of Newfoundland, complying with this Code remains voluntary. This means that each dairy producer can treat their cows as they see fit. It is impossible to distinguish a carton of milk from cows treated in accordance with the Code from one that comes from abused cows. The only obligations the industry has to meet deal with food safety.

Stretching the Definition of Welfare

To be blunt, most often, when we improve the comfort of cows, it's not so much to reduce their suffering but to increase productivity. Federations defend the rights of producers, not of animals.

Here is a simple example to show that, for the industry, the definition of animal welfare is elastic. In October 2011, the theme of the thirty-fifth annual symposium on dairy cattle was "Seizing Opportunities to Be Cost-effective!" Between a presentation titled "How to Use Genomics to Maximize Profits for Dairy Farms" and another on "Reducing Labor Costs," you could attend a speech on "Improving the Welfare of Cows to Increase Profitability on Dairy Farms."[9] In his presentation, "Comfortably Milk!", Michel Lemire, a dairy farmer from Saint-Zéphirin-de-Courval, explained how a few simple measures increased the productivity of his farm, which now ranks among the best in Quebec.

Lemire added fluorescent lights, changed his ventilation system, and moved the tie rail to give cows more space so they can "stand up without hitting the bar, which prevents the development of a lump on the neck over time."[10] A higher tie rail, however, requires a slightly longer chain, as the producer acknowledged: "The cows' heads were hanging in the air and they could not lie down on their sides." So the chains were extended from 61 to 91 cm. But not for all cows. Indeed, this new "freedom" was causing complications during milking—the more nervous ones increasingly tried to get away, and the ones in heat rubbed themselves against the milking operator! Lemire therefore solved the problem by shortening their chains "for a certain period of time."

Lemire is surely a good, conscientious producer who loves his animals; he proudly presented the results of his most recent changes. Since he was invited to go on stage, he must be exemplary—a model of best practices. But if these practices suffice to increase profits, we are still far from optimal treatment with regard to the welfare of cows.

Dairy producers are smart. They know that their animals need much more than new neon lights or longer chains. When I asked one of them why he didn't send his cows outside, he shrugged and said that his productivity would decrease: "Our margins are so low, I can't afford to do that." As long as the law fails to regulate farm practices, the improvements to conditions for animals will have only one objective: to produce more at the lowest possible cost.

What happens when the consumer pays more for organic milk, cheese, or yogurt, for example? As we will see in the next chapter, this in no way guarantees that the cows have been treated better.

8

CHEESE IS GREEN

Are certified organic dairy products better? They don't contain antibiotics and the animals are fed pesticide-free grain. They may also come from local farms with a more humane scale. However, the difference between organic and traditional milk is marginal in terms of animal welfare. As for the environmental impact, cheese, like meat, is a major source of greenhouse gases. It would be greener to abstain from animal products one day per week than to be a locavore a hundred percent of the time!

"I'M TWENTY-SIX YEARS OLD, I work full-time as a journalist for *Le Soleil* and I live with three roommates in the Saint-Jean-Baptiste district of Quebec City. The ideal circumstances for neglecting my diet . . . and my ecological footprint." Having made this lucid observation, Marc Allard decided to challenge himself. Over thirty days, he would put his environmentalist values into practice and try to reduce his footprint on the planet.

In the fall of 2008, he posted a journal entry every day, inviting readers to provide comments and encouragement.

He made himself broccoli for lunch and cabbage for dinner. He bought nothing new and ate organic food.

One of his first surprises was the fact that organic milk costs twice what regular milk does. But Allard believed that paying more meant he was buying milk that was produced using better methods. A reader set him straight: "The difference between organic and conventional milk is not that big [. . .] . I don't know one milk producer in the province who doesn't feed grass to his cows, and manure and slurry are always put back in the fields as fertilizer, regardless of the method."[1] How was that possible?

As a good journalist, Allard wanted to know the whole story. He decided to go see for himself how organic and regular milk are made. His first stop was the Pérou farm in Baie-Saint-Paul, which produces conventional milk. Tied in stalls, the cows never went outside, even in summer. The owner, Richard Bouchard, explained that it was for their own good: "This is why when we built here, we gave them as much comfort as possible."[2]

Allard took to the road again and three hours later arrived at the Optimus organic farm in Lotbinière. He felt a sense of déjà vu. What was the difference between this farm and the conventional one? "I expected to see a different setting, perhaps a little more bucolic [. . .] . The barn was almost identical. Cows tied in stalls, grazing, sleeping, peeing, defecating and being milked twice a day, every morning and evening. A mechanical system removes manure, which is stored in airtight containers and reused as fertilizer. The same kinds of milking machines and sanitary equipment are used."

Organic Is Green (But Not Necessarily Better for Animals)

Are organic and conventional one and the same? No, because there are some differences. But these lie mainly in the way grains used for animal feed are cultivated rather than in the treatment of animals. In organic milk production, the grain, grass, and hay that are given to cows must be produced organically, which is to say without pesticides or chemical fertilizers. The use of genetically modified (GMO) seeds is also prohibited. This is indeed a good thing for the environment. But it's still a far cry from a cow frolicking in the fields, followed closely by her calf still unsteady on its long spindly legs.

Genetically, organic cows are the same milk-producing machines as conventional cows. Artificial insemination is permitted and these cows also get pregnant while they are still producing milk. More importantly, their babies are taken away from them at birth just the same. Like in the conventional sector, males are auctioned to become meat. As for the females, they aren't much luckier. As the Canada Organic Agriculture Centre reports, "On many organic farms there is little difference in approach between the methods used to rear dairy calves and those used on non-organic farms."[3] Mastitis, an inflammation of the udder that causes cows so much suffering, is about as common in the organic sector as in the traditional one.[4]

In other words, in terms of the cows' welfare, the difference is very subtle. Organic certification rules allow lactating cows to move a little bit—they must have access to grazing land during summer, and in winter they must exercise at least twice a week.[5] However, at the end of their lives, organic cull cows suffer the same fate as their cousins. They go through the same auctions and endure the same endless journeys in cattle trucks, then die in the same slaughterhouses.[6] And their flesh will be mixed with that of conventional cows in the same ground beef patties.

Is Dairy Production Harmful to the Environment?

We've heard a lot about "Meatless Mondays."[7] In recent years, many people have reduced their meat consumption for environmental reasons. Since the publication, in 2006, of a UN report indicating that 18 percent of greenhouse gas emissions are attributable to livestock,[8] steaks and Hummers have become somewhat synonymous. Admittedly, habits take time to change. But it's becoming increasingly difficult to be green while in the same breath defending one's right to eat steak at all costs. But we're talking about meatless Mondays, not cheeseless Mondays. Some well-intentioned people are substituting their meat with other animal protein—like cheese. Is this better? What are the environmental effects of milk production?

After the publication of my first book, I was invited by a group of students to lecture on the ecological impact of our food choices. My presentation was scheduled at the end of a day of workshops on the environment and was preceded by a cocktail reception. I was looking forward to it—nothing better than a glass of white wine before speaking publicly.

However, when the time came, I was quite surprised to see that it wasn't a cocktail reception, but a wine-and-cheese affair. While leaving my things at the coatcheck, I saw one of the organizers and shared my uneasiness with him.

Eating Organic in Figures

Eating organic comes with a price. In Quebec grocery stores, while a two-liter container of 2% milk sells for less than $4, certified organic costs $2 more.

"Cheese at an environmental event? That strikes me as a curious choice. Especially since what I'm going to tell you in about ten minutes' time might take away your appetite."

"Oh, so you're vegan? We have grapes, too."

"No, that's not the problem. It's just that in terms of carbon emissions, it's hard to do worse than cheese. . . ."

"It's organic, no problem."

"Hmm. . . . I do hope you'll stay for my presentation."

Calculations are complex and studies are expensive, but we have more and more data measuring the carbon emissions of different foods throughout their life cycle: from the farm to the fork, including processing and transportation. In 2011, an Environmental Working Group team published a report with the greenhouse gas emissions for various protein sources.[9] The amount of CO_2 emitted was compared for each kilogram of food. Not surprisingly, meats were on the winners' podium, with lamb and beef taking the gold and silver medals. But what do we find in third place, ahead of pork, salmon, turkey, and chicken? Cheese.

Blame It on Cheese

For every kilogram of cheese produced, 13.5 kg of CO_2 are emitted into the atmosphere. This is as much as an 80-km

**Figure 8:1. Total Greenhouse Gas Emissions
from Various Proteins and Vegetables[10]**

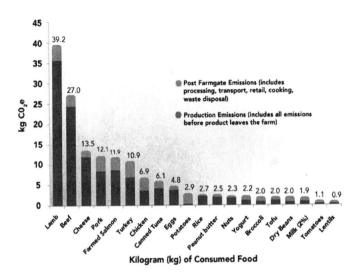

Kilogram (kg) of Consumed Food

trip by car.[11] It's hard to believe that cheese production can pollute that much. How can this be? First, we must take into account the production of the grain that is fed to cows. It requires chemical fertilizers, pesticides, and machinery, which are dependent on fossil fuels and produce greenhouse gases. Then, we must remember that cows, when digesting, emit a greenhouse gas—methane. Finally, milk must be processed into cheese. On average, 10 kg of milk are needed to manufacture one kg of cheese. This step also requires energy, but the amount varies from one cheese to another: the ones that are ripened less consume less energy. Similarly, softer and less dense cheeses—like cottage cheese—will have a smaller energy footprint because they require less milk and a shorter ripening process. Obviously, transportation must also be taken into account. Imported cheeses that are shipped by air emit on average 46 percent more CO_2 than the ones manufactured locally. However, shipping by boat has virtually no impact on the energy footprint.[12]

These statistics are calculated using factory farm data from Wisconsin, the top-ranking U.S. state when it comes to making cheese. But what about a small local producer who lets his animals go outside? Unfortunately, it doesn't make much difference. Indeed, grazing cows also emit methane, and small cheese production requires as much energy as industrial production (if not more, since the latter allows for economies of scale). What about goat cheese? It's equivalent, say the researchers.[13]

What about Other Dairy Products?

Other dairy products have much smaller carbon footprints than cheese. For instance, one kg of yogurt produces only 2.2 kg of CO_2 and one kg of milk less than two kg of CO_2, which is slightly less than one kg of broccoli. Furthermore, a study published in 2010 compared the nutrition densities of different beverages and looked at how these figures related to CO_2 emissions. Milk ended up having the best ratio, followed by orange juice and soymilk (water and soft drinks obviously have almost no footprint, but then, they're also not really nutritious!).[14]

The fact remains that the sum total of the dairy sector (milk, butter, cream, yogurt, and cheese) accounts for about four percent of all anthropogenic greenhouse gas emissions, according to the FAO.[15] This figure includes emissions related to the production, processing, and transportation of milk products as well as those related to the production of meat from animals of the dairy sector. A team from the École Polytechnique in Montreal estimated with even more precision that, in 2006, the Canadian dairy industry emitted the equivalent of 9,247,632 tonnes of CO_2. This is much more than the whole airline industry (6.2 million tonnes) or mining industry (eight million tonnes).[16]

Cow's Milk Is Thirsty

The last time I was in San Francisco, I noticed that most cafes had posted signs reading "Serious water problems. Water served on request." The drought problem in California is a serious one and there's no doubt that having restaurants try to do their part is a good thing, but I cannot help wondering what the behavioral effect of a sign like that is. Not drinking water while we eat may help us forget the inconvenient truth that agriculture accounts for between 80 and 90 percent of the fresh water used in the United States,[17] and that at least half of that goes to raising and feeding farmed animals.[18] Media often point the finger at almonds, which are indeed a very thirsty crop. But forage and alfalfa, commodities grown almost exclusively to feed beef and dairy cattle, use about four times as much water as almonds.

A recent study published in the journal *Ecological Indicators* compared the water footprints of soymilk and cow's milk and found that the water footprint of one liter of cow's milk is more than three times that of soymilk: 1,050 liters compared to is 297 liters.[19]

When will we be seeing signs saying "Serious water problems. Lattes now served with soymilk"?

Should an Ecologist Be Locavore or Veggie?

As part of his thirty-day challenge, the journalist Marc Allard tried to eat local: he only consumed foods produced within a hundred miles of his home. He even refused to eat potatoes cultivated in the Lake Saint-Jean region, less than 250 km away! His experiment is part of a trend that began in California in the early 2000s: locavorism, or only eating food that is produced locally in order to reduce CO_2 emissions from transportation and to support the local economy.

A highlight of Allard's experience was the delivery of his first local organic food basket. What did it contain? Vegetables, but also meat. "I don't know yet what the heck I'll do with that rutabaga, butternut squash, red cabbage and, oh my god, pink radish (any suggestions?). On the other hand, as a dedicated carnivore, I already dream about pork strips and head cheese, not to mention bison steak. All organic, of course."[20] But in reality, is it better to be vegan or locavore?

Although most environmental campaigns focus on buying local, it is by reducing our consumption of animal products that we can have the greatest positive impact on the environment. In fact, transportation is estimated to count for only 11 percent of greenhouse gas emissions related to food. Recent studies show that from an environmental point of view, we have a greater impact by being vegan (that is to say, eating no meat, no dairy, and no eggs) even just one day a week, rather than being locavore seven days a week.[21] If he'd have agreed to make a few sacrifices in terms of his meat consumption, Marc Allard could have indulged in some exotic fruits or nuts for lunch while reducing his environmental footprint. He could even have afforded to consume several pounds of Lake Saint-Jean potatoes!

The idea that replacing beef or poultry with cheese is an eco-friendly move is therefore misguided. As is celebrating our environmental consciousness with a plate of organic cheeses. The problem is that cheese is everywhere. And it's everywhere because it is produced by an industry that is not quite like any other.

9

IT'S AN INDUSTRY JUST LIKE ANY OTHER

The dairy industry is an industry like no other. Consumers have an emotional attachment to dairy farmers, and the dairy industry also represents a powerful lobby. Over time, this lobby has set up the mechanisms required to ensure economic stability. The industry escapes the usual rules of supply and demand, but that doesn't stop it from being one of the country's biggest advertisers.

OUR IMAGINATION DIVIDES THE WORLD into good guys and bad guys—and farmers and traditional values fall on the good side. We feel a certain affection for farmers and trust them completely, as a survey conducted in 2010 by Léger Marketing showed. To the question, "What professions do you trust the most?" Quebecers first mentioned firefighters, followed by nurses, mail carriers, doctors, optometrists . . . and farmers. Even before teachers, opticians, and electricians![1] We trust them, and can also easily identify with them. Barely fifty years ago, the province of Quebec was still a basically rural society imbued with values connected to the land. Everyone has a farmer in their family. Agriculture remains a big source of pride for Quebec, an important part of the province's social and cultural imagination.

Of the whole farming profession, dairy farmers are probably the ones we admire most. They are the "real" farmers—hard workers living on small family farms, with children who don't mind pitching in. Milk is a product of *our* land and promotes *our* values. Our attachment to the land is what makes the dairy industry an industry like no other.

Figure 9:1. Dairy Farms and Cows by Canadian Province, 2012

Province	Dairy Farms	Lactating Cows	Cows per Farm
Quebec	6,281	368,000	59
Ontario	4,137	322,900	78
Alberta	592	90,000	152
British Columbia	512	71,500	140
Manitoba	344	44,500	129
Nova Scotia	245	21,800	89
New Brunswick	219	18,700	85
Prince Edward Island	200	13,200	66
Saskatchewan	182	29,000	159
Newfoundland	34	5,700	168
Total	12,746	985,300	77

But beyond the stereotypical image of the country farmer with his rubber boots, the dairy industry also seeks to protect its own interests and maximize profits. It fights to maintain its current level of revenues and promotes consumption of its products. It's even one of the country's most powerful lobbies and has managed to make milk a unique product that's exempt from the usual market forces.

Promoting Stability

Founded in 1934, the Dairy Farmers of Canada association has a clear mission: "DFC strives to create stable conditions for the Canadian dairy industry, today and in the future. It works to maintain policies that foster the viability of Canadian dairy farmers and promote dairy products and their health benefits."[2] The key word here is *stability*. The dairy sector escapes the usual trade rules. DFC has succeeded where no other private sector has before it: it created a market closed to foreign competition. When DFC talks stability, it means the guarantee of a regular income.

Supply Management

To achieve this stability in income, dairy farmers have established a very special mechanism that's unlike any other in the world: supply management. The idea is to adjust production and use collective marketing to meet the domestic demand without the need for a free market.

One of the main arguments in favor of this mechanism is that it ensures a good balance between supply and demand. Thus, before the introduction of this program in the 1970s, the market was free: each dairy farm owner produced as much as he or she wanted. This would inevitably lead to a glut and the plummeting of prices paid to producers. Supply management restored some balance. There is no longer any overproduction, and prices are stable. The mechanism was then also implemented by the producers of both poultry and eggs. In total, 20 percent of Canadian agricultural products are made within the supply management system.[3]

Two organizations are responsible for everything related to supply management. At the federal level, they are concerned with the amount of milk that will be processed into cheese and other products (60 percent of the total), while the provinces manage fluid milk. A quota system establishes the expected monthly production based on estimates of the market demand. These quotas are somewhat comparable to the "rights to produce" purchased by dairy producers. No quota, no dairy farm. This means that the industry is protected by a barrier to entry. One simply doesn't become a dairy farmer just like that, buying cows and selling milk. One must first and foremost purchase a quota from a farmer who is willing to sell it, and find the money to do this.

And this is one of this system's main problems. The costs of quotas are high: about $25,000 per cow.[4] Getting into this industry means being in debt for a few decades. In return, the quota guarantees a stable income. The price paid to the producer is set by the Canadian Dairy Commission, which establishes it objectively, taking into account production costs (it corresponds on average to 50 percent of the price consumers pay at the grocery store).[5] Farmers then sell their milk to a union that markets and distributes it. In Quebec, this is the role of the Quebec Federation of Milk Producers (FPLQ), which is affiliated with a professional farmers' union, the Union des Producteurs Agricoles (UPA).

In addition, high tariffs are imposed on dairy products imported into the country. They vary from 202 percent for skim milk to 298 percent for butter; the taxes levied on cheese, yogurt, ice cream, and whole milk are in the same range.[6] Imported products are thus very expensive, which clearly benefits the domestic market.

Our dairy producers are afraid of globalization and the international agreements signed by our governments—they fear that these may jeopardize their supply management system and protected market. They repeatedly demand the help and protection of various levels of government.

Fixed Prices

Grocers are free to set the prices of the lettuce, cereal, or ham they sell as they wish. But not the price of milk. In Quebec, the retail price for a liter of milk is established by the Agricultural Marketing Board (Régie des Marchés Agricoles et Alimentaires), and this has been the case since 1935. The Board actually sets a minimum and maximum price for fluid milk that retailers must abide by. You will never see milk for $0.50 per liter at Costco.

Milk Production in Quebec: Key Figures

There are about 6,300 dairy farms in Quebec; this figure represents nearly half of all Canadian farms.[7] In 2009, milk production created nearly 25,000 direct jobs, and processing operations, about 8,500.[8] If the dairy industry were a single company, it would rank among the largest employers in the province of Quebec. (The biggest employer, Desjardins Group, totals 39,000 employees, and the number two, Metro, 32,000.[9])

You might think that such a practice benefits consumers by guaranteeing them cheap milk, but some analysts have voiced doubts. Sylvain Charlebois of the University of Guelph is of the opinion that the price is established unilaterally. "It takes into account the production, distribution, and retail market costs of milk, but it doesn't factor in consumers' ability to pay."[10] The law also favors certain industries at the expense of buyers. Indeed, the price of milk is determined by the way it will be used. Frozen pizza preparation facilities, for instance, are granted a special permit from the government that enables them to buy cheese at a lower cost than pizzerias,[11] a practice condemned by restaurant owners, who recently launched a campaign for deregulation of the price of milk.[12]

An exception is the so-called "value-added" milks. This term refers to any milk that is not sold in a carton or bag. This largely explains dairy producers' interest in all types of flavored or long-life milks, which now account for 45 percent of sales.[13]

Protected Designation

Under the food and drug regulations, the term "milk" is protected—it can be used only to refer to "the normal lacteal secretion obtained from the mammary gland of the cow." Milk from any animal other than a cow must include the name of that animal on its label. If milk is made from a plant, another designation has to be used. So you can't sell soy *milk*—it has to be called soy *beverage*. And yet, for some reason, no one is calling for coconut milk to be renamed!

Milk It

In 2010, Quebecers spent more than $2 billion on fresh dairy products. This represents 15 percent of their total grocery spending.[14] While many industries are suffering from the financial crisis, dairy farmers can be glad that their market

Got Milk?

American producers contribute to the "National Dairy Checkoff" at the rate of fifteen cents per hundredweight of milk.[15] Ten cents of this goes to the regional checkoff, while the other five cents goes to the national checkoff.[16] The money is used for generic promotion of dairy products, new product development, and nutrition education.

In 1995, the U.S. government created Dairy Management Inc., a nonprofit corporation with the mission of increasing dairy consumption by "offering the products consumers want, where and when they want them." Dairy Managements' annual budget of about $136 million is largely paid for by the National Dairy Checkoff. In comparison, the Center for Nutrition Policy and Promotion, which promotes healthy diets, has a budget of only $6.5 million.[17]

With its "Got Milk?" campaign, Dairy Management has been successful at slowing down the decline in milk consumption, in particular by focusing on schoolchildren. It has also relentlessly marketed cheese though partnerships with fast food chains.[18]

is relatively stable. This doesn't mean the industry is not changing, however. A decline in milk consumption has been observed, although it is offset by increased sales of cheese and yogurt.

A \$2-billion market for dairy products obviously means that quite a few consumers have been milked: this is the same order of magnitude as the entire Canadian television and film market. In this context, influencing consumers is crucial. As indicated in Figure 9:3 (on page 125), the advertising expenditures for dairy products account for nearly 30 percent of the total amount invested in the promotion of food and non-alcoholic beverages in Canada.[19] The Canadian dairy industry invests over \$1 billion in advertising annually— almost half of the amount spent by all mobile phone companies combined. Comparisons with other types of food are even more striking. The promotion of fruit and vegetables accounts for only six percent of ad spending, which is similar to the figures for other animal proteins.

Approximately 15 percent of these expenditures are made directly by associations of dairy producers. The remaining 85 percent are incurred by large processors to market their different brands: Agropur, Parmalat, and Saputo. Finally, it is interesting to note that cheese is the item for which the most advertising investments are made in Canada, with 42 percent of dairy farmers' advertising budget allocated to this product alone.[20]

Supply management thus truly makes the Canadian dairy industry an industry like no other. It's hard to say whether this is good or bad from an economic point of view. However, it probably has consequences for animal welfare because the only way milk producers can increase their revenues is to reduce costs. No wonder, then, that they are reluctant to lengthen the chains that keep their cows in their stalls. For a dairy farmer, the equation is a simple one: if expenses increase, earnings decrease. If cows are allowed to go out of the barn and their productivity decreases, the farmer loses revenues.

Finally, the dairy industry is not an industry like any other mainly because the raw material involved is not like any other. Cows may be the means of production, but they cannot be just that. They are also living beings who deserve some respect. However, the industry sells us milk as if it were an ordinary commodity, not much different from fruit juice, just another normal product. Philosophers sometimes ask what kinds of items should be excluded from economic markets. After all, most people would agree that blood or human organs should not be bought or sold, because they are not commodities. I don't know if milk should be classified in that category. But I do know that trading in the mass exploitation of conscious, non-consenting sentient beings can never be an industry just like any other.

Figure 9:2. Advertising Expenditures in Canada for Dairy Products
(2011) Source: Nielson, 2011

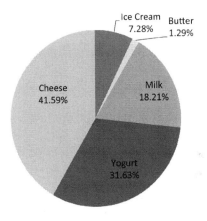

Figure 9:3. Advertising Expenditures in Canada for Food and
Drinks (excluding alcohol) (2011) Source: Nielson, 2011

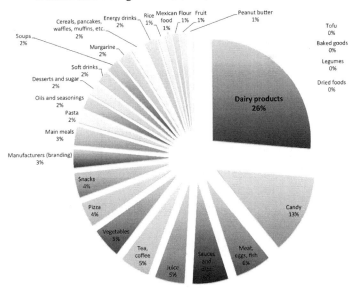

10

I COULD NEVER LIVE WITHOUT CHEESE

Cheese seems to have a special power to make us love it. Humans have innate predispositions making us crave fat and foods with rich and exciting flavors. Furthermore, cheese is said to contain various compounds from the morphine family. But as with any addiction, you can learn to do without it.

A FRIEND HAS JUST SHARED her despair about the acne taking over her face with her friends on Facebook. "Ultimatum to my face: I'm beginning to seriously consider Accutane." Since we're on Facebook, I reply with a few links. And since I'm a little obsessed with this topic, these links go to studies on dairy consumption and hormonal problems, including acne. I also suggest that as a test, she could stop eating dairy products for a few weeks. To see what happens.

"Does that mean cutting cheese out, too?" she asks.

"Yes, of course," I reply.

"Even goat cheese?"

"Well, yes."

"No way I could ever do that."

Like most of us, my friend is sure she couldn't do without cheese. Cutting out meat, eggs, or milk? Sure, why not? But cheese? Impossible. Even though we have very good reasons to stop eating cheese (health, ecology, and animal ethics), it seems to be the most difficult thing to leave out of our diet. That's what I thought myself a few years ago. Although I am now quite used to finishing a bottle of wine without a piece of bread topped with runny blue cheese, I still occasionally have cheese cravings. What's going on?

The Force of Habit

We don't really choose what we eat and we don't choose to love cheese. Of course, at a restaurant or grocery store, we show our preference for one type of food or another. But basically, we have innate predispositions that result in our choices being already made before we have actually chosen. A preference for fat and sugar, for example, is universal.

Indeed, psychologist Paul Rozin explains how our biological predispositions evolved in an environment that is completely different from the one we know today.[1] Our Pleistocene hunter-gatherer ancestors (between 2.5 million years ago and 10,000 BCE) lived in a world where food was scarce and not very diverse. The foods they found contained little fat or sugar. They had to work hard to be able to eat, and their life expectancy was short. If there was a chance to eat a fatty piece of meat or a sweet fruit, they would never think twice, since their survival depended on it. Evolution thus selected for tastes suited to this type of environment. Our taste preferences are the same as those of our hunter-gatherer ancestors.

Today, the situation is obviously quite different—to find fat or sugar, all we have to do is go to the store. However, we still have just about the same taste buds and brains as our ancestors. We still have this insatiable appetite for fatty and sugary foods, even though we don't really need them anymore.

Cheese is high in fat. In 100 g of cheddar, there are 30 g of fat. In this sense, it is "natural" for Westerners to love cheese and it greatly appeals to our palate. This also explains why we are not that passionate for green vegetables, which are much more abundant in nature. But preferring or craving a certain food doesn't mean it's what's best for our health.

A Matter of Smell

It goes without saying that we like food that tastes good. But the flavor of food does not come from what our taste buds perceive. Rather, we detect a food's flavor by breathing in its scent. Without realizing it, when we chew and swallow, we send small fragrant puffs to the back of our mouths and into our nasal passages. The smell of food therefore overshadows what we perceive with our taste buds. In fact, our sense of taste is very basic. We can distinguish only five tastes: sweet, salty, sour, bitter, and umami. Everything else stems from the scents perceived by our retronasal tract.

In *Neurogastronomy: How the Brain Creates Flavor and Why It Matters*,[2] neurobiologist Gordon M. Shepherd describes how our olfactory sense works. He explains, for example, that for every flavor our brain constructs complex images. These are associated with emotions, which play an important role in our motivation to perform actions. In particular, these emotions cause us to make great efforts to get certain foods. (It is also worth noting that the word "emotion" comes from the Latin *motio*, meaning "motion, movement, the act of moving.")

We are naturally attracted to foods with rich flavors—it is known that boring diets stimulate cravings for foods with more exciting flavors.[3] That's why replacing cheese with plain tofu is unlikely to satisfy our neurons. This explains, in short, the sense of deprivation we feel when we remove cheese from our diet.

Morphine in Cheese?

Just like with caffeine, nicotine, and alcohol, it's possible to become addicted to some common foods like cheese. Indeed, cheese's complex flavor can be addictive, but it is also said to contain various compounds from the morphine family. It has been known for some years that the fermentation required to produce cheese is a source of casomorphins,[4] proteins that have analgesic properties similar to those of morphine. Digesting milk also produces casomorphins— casein, the main protein found in milk, is destroyed during this process and releases amino acids that group into chains of casomorphins. Finally, milk contains small quantities of "pure" morphine produced naturally by cows.[5] And morphine means addiction. Dr. Neal Barnard, author of *Breaking the Food Seduction*,[6] sees this as one of the main causes of our infatuation with cheese.

It should be noted, however, that opinions are divided on this issue. In a report published in 2009, the European Food Safety Authority (EFSA) said it didn't have sufficient evidence to take a position on the ability of casomorphins to pass through the intestinal wall, enter the bloodstream, and finally cross the blood–brain barrier.[7]

From Asceticism to Veganism

When we look at the history of veganism—the diet in which the consumption of all animal products is avoided—we can see that we've been addicted to cheese (and milk) for ages. While it seems likely that there have always been vegetarian humans, traces of veganism are much harder to find. So who were the first humans to give up cheese? That's exactly the question I asked Renan Larue, historian of vegetarianism.[9]

Addiction: Not Only Physical

Being addicted to a certain food doesn't mean we have to go through a withdrawal period with tremors and dry mouth symptoms if we decide to stop consuming it. As Dr. Neal Barnard sees it, addiction to a food product is similar to a gambling addiction: the person has a compulsive need to play, and may even be willing to take risks to do so, but does not necessarily feel any physical withdrawal symptoms when the casino is closed. Similarly, one can be addicted to cheese without necessarily having cold sweats when the tray is empty.[8]

Whether the addiction is psychological or physical, the substance stimulates the brain's opiate receptors, creating a little buzz. As soon as addiction sets in, the brain expects the stimulation to continue.

"In the long history of vegetarianism, it is essentially meat that received the strongest criticism from vegetarians," he replied. "Abstaining from milk in addition to meat seems to be primarily associated with religious and philosophical groups that follow a different principle: asceticism. In the West, veganism was until very recently seen as an extreme practice, an exercise in penitential discipline." Indeed, not that long ago, giving up dairy products was a way to sacrifice physical pleasures in general to achieve spiritual betterment. Some religious people today do adopt a vegan diet during the "fasting" days of the liturgical calendar.

If we set aside religious practices and examine ethical considerations, we can see that cow's milk has long been a reason for being vegetarian, not vegan. As Larue explains, "since Antiquity, proponents of vegetarianism have emphasized the services that cows—these innocent creatures—perform for us so as to better highlight the cruelty and ingratitude of those who put them to death. For them, the milk we get from the cows should compel us, in turn, to respect them, which is to say, to not eat them. Our benevolence towards them is a debt repaid, a kind of contractual obligation."

To be able to imagine living without animals, humans first had to develop the technology to do so. Throughout Antiquity, there were no tractors or chemical fertilizers, so we were dependent on the driving force of cattle. At that time, a human society without cows was not even a utopia— it was something nobody had thought of! The only possible solution, the best we could offer animals, was vegetarianism, and treating them with respect.

Today, the situation is different. The idea that we can live without eating or exploiting animals, although still marginal, is becoming more widespread. The term *vegan* originated in England in the mid-twentieth century after members of the Vegetarian Society suggested forming a group of vegetarians who did not consume dairy products (or eggs). The Vegan Society was founded in 1944. Even today, it defines veganism as a lifestyle that seeks to exclude, as far as possible, all forms of animal exploitation and cruelty, whether for food, clothing, or any other purpose.[10] For many vegans, this choice is nothing more than the logical culmination of the commitment vegetarianism is based on.

Cheese, Please!

Vegans are still a minority and the dairy industry doesn't plan on giving up its profits. The industry has also realized that we really love cheese. Dr. Neal Barnard tells how Dairy Management Inc., the U.S. equivalent of the Dairy Farmers of Canada, supported the development of Pizza Hut's "Ultimate Cheese Lover's" pizza with a cheese-stuffed crust. The same organization also worked with Burger King to ensure that cheese is included in all their burgers.[11]

In Quebec, the ad campaign promoting local cheeses was— and still is—meant to develop an attachment to cheese that is not only physical, but also emotional. It is now Quebecers' favorite local food, before strawberries, apples, and maple syrup.[12] While milk and ice cream sales have been declining for years, cheese sales are in full swing. From 10.45 kg per capita per year in 1990, the average Canadian consumed 12.54 kg cheese in 2010, which fell slightly to 12.02 kg in 2014.[13]

Figure 10:1. Consumption of Dairy Products
Per Capita, Per Year (Canada)

	1990	2000	2010
Milk (l)	95.47	88.22	77.98
Cream (l)	5.25	6.83	8.21
Yogurt (l)	2.91	4.59	8.28
Ice Cream (l)	10.51	8.63	5.51
Butter (kg)	2.71	2.99	2.69
Cheese (kg)	10.45	11.85	12.54

Changing Habits

Whether for health or ethical reasons, shifting away from a cheese addiction is not an easy task. Following are a few tips to help you in your transition.

Our relationship with food is largely social. By trying to change your eating habits with someone—a spouse, a friend, a child—you multiply your chances of success.

- Your friends may question your choice, and that's perfectly normal. It is indeed natural and even beneficial to be careful with dietary changes. When a baby chimp grabs a fruit that is not commonly eaten in his community, his mother or sister will take it away from him as a precaution. This does not mean that the fruit is poisonous, but that they prefer to avoid taking the risk. Friends and family members often have the same kind of reaction when we announce that we have changed our diet. It's because they care about us.
- If you have decided to stop consuming dairy products, don't make a cheesy dish for the rest of your family.

Instead, offer to share your cheese-free meal with them. We often strive to cook what pleases others to show them that we love them. But preparing healthy meals is also a good way to show our love!

- Talk about it! When I decided to give up dairy products, I was a bit embarrassed to tell my co-workers about it. Today, I regret this. Once I finally did explain the motivations behind my choice, most people showed support. Often, before choosing a place for lunch, they would ask me if I would be able to find something to eat there. The same principle applies when we are invited to eat at someone's home. We can opt to make exceptions, but we can also choose to help the host or hostess prepare dishes that are compatible with our diet.

- Don't say you'll never eat cheese again. Give yourself the right to "cheat." The goal is to do your best. Not to be perfect![14]

- Talk about other things! Your dietary change may fascinate people, but it can sometimes be tiring to have to explain the reasons behind your choices over and over again. Your food choices are personal. You don't have to become an anti-milk activist and never talk about anything else!

CONCLUSION

I HAVE DEDICATED THIS BOOK to a cow. A Jersey cow bearing the number 67—a beautiful brunette with dark eyes and delicate eyelashes, like the Greek goddess Hera. I crossed paths with Jersey cow no. 67 a few months ago at a farm show. She caught my eye because, unlike the other cows, who were rather quiet that day, she refused to walk in step with the rest. She pulled on her rope and did not seem to fear the blows raining down on her flanks from a wooden stick. She pulled on the rope and refused to move. I stopped to watch her because she stood out. That's when, in the middle of this farm show, a simple question hit me: What was she doing there?

This Jersey cow was there because we believe it's natural to drink cow's milk. However, milk consumption is recent, dating only from the beginnings of agriculture, about ten thousand years ago. Furthermore, humans had to evolve the necessary adaptations to be able to consume cow's milk—one of our genes had to mutate so we could digest it. Today, it is mainly the descendants of Europeans or African nomadic peoples who can digest it in adulthood. This small group accounts for barely 25 percent of the world's population.

This Jersey cow was there because we believe that her milk is necessary for healthy bones and preventing osteoporosis. But milk isn't what we need to grow strong bones. What we need is calcium, and there are numerous plant-based sources of this nutrient, as well as vitamin D and a healthy lifestyle. Cow's milk is not only far from essential—it also contains hormones, allergens, cholesterol, saturated fat, casomorphins, and pesticides that are harmful to our health.

Another reason this Jersey cow was there is that the industry is funding research aimed at convincing us of the necessity and advantages of drinking milk. She was there because we're willing to ignore the fact that her cheese significantly contributes to global warming. She was there because dairy producers invest in advertising campaigns to make us love her milk and cheese. She was there because our relationship with dairy products is based on myths in which facts are denied in favor of our own pleasure.

Jersey cow no. 67 and the millions of her fellow cows who stand in stables are there only for our pleasure. They are there because we find it convenient to use them for their milk before killing them for meat. But we should never forget that cows produce milk only because we force them to. They spend most of their lives tied in their stalls, constantly pregnant, and separated from their calves just after giving birth. Reduced to simple machines that convert fodder and soymeal into money, their only future is the slaughterhouse, after four years of misery. They suffer physically and psychologically, but no law protects them. Basically, this Jersey cow was there only because we're very good at forgetting about her pain while we eat our cereal.

How can something be natural, necessary, and normal when we have the horrible feeling that it is not?

* * *

I can't think of any moral justification for our consumption of cow's milk. People who are familiar with my work know that I've been vegan for several years now. They're also aware that, like everyone else, I was originally an omnivore—and a carnist without knowing it! I then embraced a kind of "semi-vegetarianism" (I was still eating fish) and then full vegetarianism. Finally, I realized that the arguments against meat applied to all foods of animal origin. Maintaining the status quo was impossible. The decision to become vegan first seemed quite extreme to me; today, I realize that it was reasonable, since I was only aligning my actions with my knowledge.

Changing habits is not easy, and you may need to proceed slowly and go through a number of steps. However, in light of what I now know about dairy, I wonder if we should not approach these steps differently. Why not consider starting with "semi-veganism"? We could reduce our consumption of both meat and dairy products at the same time. In many ways, this might be a better compromise than regular vegetarianism. Perhaps our society could, in addition to Meatless Mondays, promote Dairy-free Tuesdays.

Animal ethics arguments really resonate with me, and I'm of the opinion that we should attempt to live without causing unnecessary suffering. I know we can prepare and enjoy vegan meals without ever missing butter or juicy steaks; it can even become a creative and delicious experience on an equal footing with the best culinary traditions. Above all, even if perfection seems unattainable and a life without animal protein seems utopian, that doesn't mean it's not worth trying. I know we can enjoy life without innocent sentient beings having to pay the price for it.

I hope I have shown that when it comes to animal ethics and environmental protection, the dairy industry doesn't have the best record. But as I was writing this book, I also learned things I hadn't even imagined, like the negative impact milk consumption has on human health. Many studies link milk consumption to health problems to varying degrees including allergic reactions, various cancers, heart disease, and obesity.

Admittedly, milk is not a poison. But it is not an essential food either. Human beings are not somehow the only mammal that, once weaned, still depends on the mammary glands of another animal for survival. Unlike what the industry would have us believe, we *can* live without milk. We can live perfectly well without it, and maybe even better. Milk is not the miraculous beverage they're making it out to be.

* * *

No doubt about it—our habits are deeply ingrained. And we can count on the dairy industry to further complicate our task and perpetuate myths. Millions of dollars are spent on advertising campaigns that monopolize television airwaves and newspaper space. Very intelligent people are hired to think about the best ways to gain our sympathy, enslave our desires, and ensure that we stick with our habits. And it's true that milk ads are often quite appealing.

But that's not a good reason. We must learn to think rather than believe. We must dare to assert our own values, refuse to let others dictate our choices, and have the courage to stand out from the herd, just like Jersey cow no. 67. We must stay alert, think critically, and keep learning. This is the only way to stop being cash cows.

Appendix

Substitutes for Dairy Products

It's one thing to decide to change our habits and cut down our milk consumption. It's quite another to face the task of preparing dinner without any dairy products. Animal milk is everywhere, and in all our recipes. Replacing the cream in our coffee with a soy alternative is fairly straightforward. But what do you do when you want to bake cheese lasagna?

This book would have been incomplete without the following short and handy guide, a survival kit for people moving away from dairy. I asked MariÈve Savaria, a qualified dietitian, vegan cooking instructor and blogger, to share a few of her tips.*

Replacing Milk

Grains, Nuts and Seeds Like Their Own Kind
At most grocery stores, you can find a wide range of grain and nut milks: buckwheat, oat, barley, rice, soy, almond, etc. Their nutritional properties are discussed in Chapter 2. But

---

* MariÈve Savaria's blog (in French) can be found at brutalimentation.ca.

what do they taste like? What kinds of recipes can we use them in? A simple rule of thumb is that grains go well with their own kind.

Buckwheat pancakes are especially good when made with buckwheat milk.

Sauces and soups are often thickened with some starch or a grain (such as rice) and combine well with a soy, rice, oat, or barley beverage (opt for unsweetened versions).

Rice pudding is great when made with rice milk.

Cakes, muffins, and cookies are the perfect things to bake using almond milk.

Enhance the flavor of your oatmeal cookies, porridge, or morning cereal with some oat or barley milk.

Mission: Camouflage

In coffee or a béchamel sauce, the last thing anyone wants is the taste of the plant-based milk to be too strong. For this reason, it's best to look for a subtle, neutral flavor, like that of certain unsweetened soy or almond milks.

Sweet or Savory?

First think about what kind of food or drink you will be making with your plant-based milk. A dessert? Pasta with a tomato cream sauce? Pudding? This is what will dictate your choice of one plant-based milk over another.

Commercially Available Plant-Based Cheeses, Creams, Yogurts, Ice Creams, and Butters

New products are appearing every week at grocery stores and health food stores. Check them out! There's as much difference between a French Camembert and a spreadable cheese as between commercial plant-based cheese that's perfect for a pizza and artisanal vegan cheese made from fermented nuts. You have to give them a try!

Making Your Own Nut-Based "Dairy" Products

No need to have a cow on hand to make your own milk, cream, or cheese. All you need is a few handfuls of nuts. The process is quite simple, and the base is always the same. Just soak the nuts or seeds in water for a few hours at room temperature, then drain and rinse. Next, add some fresh water: use more water for a liquid that is similar to animal milk and less if you want a thicker consistency that resembles cream, yogurt, or cottage cheese.

All these recipes are bases that you can modify as you wish. They will keep for about four to five days when stored in a covered glass jar in the refrigerator.

Plant-Based Milk or Cream
Yields one liter of milk or 1½ cups of cream.

Soak three-quarters of a cup nuts or seeds of your choice (almonds, sesame, sunflower, walnuts, etc.) for twelve hours.

Drain, rinse and place in your blender with four cups of fresh water.

Blend for about thirty seconds or until the mixture is milky white.

Strain using a nut-milk filtration bag or a very fine sieve.

You can add a hint of honey, maple syrup, cocoa powder, or vanilla extract to flavor your beverage and obtain a result closer to commercial plant-based milks.

Plant-Based Cream

Yields 1½ cups of cream.

Soak half a cup of cashews for at least four hours at room temperature.

Drain, rinse, and place in your blender with half a cup of water and a pinch of fleur de sel. Add a little more water if needed.

Blend until smooth. Add water if necessary.

Avoid heating this cream. Add at the end of the cooking process, once the pot is removed from the heat, or pour it on top of a plate of cooked pasta as an Alfredo-style sauce. This cream is also great as a base for creamy salad dressings.

You can also sweeten this cream, add dried fruit, and freeze it. When you take it out of the freezer, just put it in your food processor and blend to make ice cream!

Plant-Based Yogurt

Soak one cup of cashews, almonds, or sunflower seeds for at least twelve hours at room temperature.

Drain, rinse, and place in your blender with one cup of water.

Blend until smooth.

Place in a large glass jar, cover with cheesecloth or a towel secured with a rubber band, and let ferment away from light for twelve hours. Refrigerate for a few hours. Strain using a drip bag for greater smoothness. The result will be a thick yogurt or spreadable cheese that can be flavored to taste (with sugar, salt, garlic, or miso) and will keep for one week in the fridge.

ACKNOWLEDGMENTS

I would first of all like to thank everyone who commented on my blog posts, asked questions after my lectures, and sent me their thoughts by email. Your input proved a great resource as I developed my ideas.

The original version of this book benefited from the invaluable comments, advice, and constructive criticism of the following people: Alexandre Simard, Amélie Piéron, Andrée-Anne Cormier, Antoine C. Dussault, Benoît Girouard, Catherine Viau, Frédéric Côté-Boudreau, Guillaume Beaulac, Jean-François Bourdeau, Jean-Philippe Royer, Marie-Claude Plourde, MariÈve Savaria, Martine Delvaux, Martin Gibert, Olivier Berreville, Renan Larue, Roméo Bouchard, Sophie Gaillard, and Valéry Giroux. I'd also like to thank Miléna Stojanac, who is simultaneously my French publisher, confidante, and scientific advisor, along with the entire Groupe Librex staff for their friendship and the trust they placed in me.

Special thanks go to Élise Bergeron, who convinced me that *Vache à lait* could thrive in an English version. I also thank my translator, Marie-Claude Plourde, and translation reviser Elisabeth Lyman for their amazing work. And I'm particularly grateful to Dany Plouffe, Jamie Berger, and Joseph Gonzales who commented on the current edition.

I thank Kara Davis and Martin Rowe at Lantern Books for giving me a unique chance to reach a wider audience and the Société de développement des entreprises culturelles (SODEC) for their crucial financial support, which made this project possible.

NOTES

(all URLs accessed July 9, 2015)

Foreword

1   Stefano Gerosa, and Jakob Skoet, "Milk Availability: Trends in Production and Demand and Medium-term Outlook" (ESA Working Paper No. 12-01 (February 2012). Food and Agriculture Organization of the United Nations Agricultural Development Economics Division (FAO ESA), http://www.fao.org/economic/esa.

2   C. L. Delgado. "Rising Consumption of Meat and Milk in Developing Countries Has Created a New Food Revolution. *Journal of Nutrition* 133 no. 11 (2003): 3907s–3910s.

3   Bob Yonkers. "Market Update: World Dairy Situation 2011 Report." International Dairy Foods Association (IDFA), November 22, 2011, http://www.idfa.org/resource-center/market-information/update-on-dairy-markets/article/2011/11/22/market-update-world-dairy-situation-2011.

4   Food and Agriculture Organization (FAO) of the United Nations Statistics Division, "Food Supply Quantity in Selected Country," http://faostat3.fao.org/home/E.

5   Gerosa and Skoet, op. cit.

6   The Nestlé Healthy Kids Global Programme, http://www.nestle.com/nutrition-health-wellness/kids-best-start/children-family/healthy-kids-programme; Tetra Laval, *Annual Report 2011/2012* [Press release]. http://tetralaval.com/

7   Nestlé, *Annual Report 2011*, http://www. nestle.com/.

8   Food & Water Watch, 2015. *Factory Farm Nation, 2015 Edition.* http://www.foodandwaterwatch.org.

9   FAO, Dairy Production and Products. Milk Production, http://
      www.fao.org/agriculture/dairy-gateway/milk-production/
      en/#.Vc3wpyxVhBe.

10   Kanpur BDS, n.d.; n.d.). Indian leather industry, http://kanpurbds.
      fibre2fashion.com/indian-leather-ind.asp; United States Department
      of Agriculture (USDA). Livestock and Poultry: World Markets and
      Trade. Retrieved from Cornell University Mann Library, http://
      usda.mannlib.cornell.edu/MannUsda/viewDocumentInfo.
      do?documentID=1488, April 17 and October 18, 2012.

11   Marina A. G. Von Keyserlingk, *et al.* "Invited Review: Sustainability
      of the US Dairy Industry" [Abstract], *Journal of Dairy Science* 96,
      no. 9: 5405–5425, 2013, http://www.journalofdairyscience.org/.

12   Pew Commission on Industrial Farm Animal Production, 2008.
      *Putting Meat on the Table: Industrial Farm Animal Production in
      America.* Pew Charitable Trusts and John Hopkins Bloomberg School
      of Public Health, http://www.ncifap.org/_images/pcifapsmry.pdf.

13   Ibid.

14   People for the Ethical Treatment of Animals (PETA) India.
      *Inside the Indian Dairy Industry: A Report on the Abuse of Cows and
      Buffaloes Exploited for Milk.* Retrieved March 25, 2013, http://www.
      happycow.net/; Tom Levitt. "Younger Generation Face Long Wait
      for Law Change on Animal Cruelty," *China Dialogue*, February 26,
      2013, http://www.chinadialogue.net.

Introduction: Natural, Necessary, and Normal

1   Michael Shermer, *The Believing Brain: From Ghosts and Gods to
      Politics and Conspiracies—How We Construct Beliefs and Reinforce
      Them as Truths* (New York: Times Books, 2011).

Chapter 1: Milk Is Natural

1   Christopher Beam, "Man's First Friend: What Was the Original
      Domesticated Animal?" *Slate*, March 6, 2009, http://www.slate.
      com/articles/news_and_politics/explainer/2009/03/mans_
      first_friend.html.

2   Ruth Bollongino et al., "Modern Taurine Cattle Descended from
      Small Number of Near-Eastern Founders," *Molecular Biology and
      Evolution*, March 14, 2012. Quoted in Duncan Geere, "Origin of

Modern Cows Traced to Single Herd," *Wired UK*, March 27, 2012, http://www.wired.com/2012/03/cattle-ox-origins.

3   Ewen Callaway, "Pottery Shards Put a Date on Africa's Dairying," *Nature.com*, June 20, 2012, http://www.nature.com/news/pottery-shards-put-a-date-on-africa-s-dairying-1.10863.

4   Ibid.

5   Physicians Committee for Responsible Medicine, "What Is Lactose Intolerance?" http://www.pcrm.org//health/diets/vegdiets/what-is-lactose-intolerance.

6   Steven R. Hertzler, RD, Bao-Chau L. Huynh, and Dennis A. Savaiano, PhD, "How Much Lactose is Low Lactose?" *Journal of the Academy of Nutrition and Dietetics* 96, no. 3 (March 1996): 243–46.

7   Université de Genève, "Sur les traces du lait et de sa digestion," http://www.unige.ch/communication/Campus/campus97/recherche2.html.

8   Deborah Valenze, *Milk: A Local and Global History* (New Haven, CT: Yale University Press, 2011), 3.

9   Sciences et Avenir, "La tolérance au lait provient des Balkans," September 2, 2009, http://www.sciencesetavenir.fr/nature-environnement/20090902.OBS9691/la-tolerance-au-lait-provient-des-balkans.html.

10 The European Union is incidentally funding a research group, the LeCHE (Lactase Persistence in the early Cultural History of Europe), dedicated to this very phenomenon.

11 Joseph Keon, *Whitewash: The Disturbing Truth About Cow's Milk and Your Health* (Gabriola Island, BC, Canada: New Society Publishers, 2010), 46.

12 Ibid., 26.

13 Melanie Joy, *Why We Love Dogs, Eat Pigs, and Wear Cows: An Introduction to Carnism* (San Francisco: Conari Press), 13.

14 Ibid., 17.

Chapter 2: A Glass of Milk for Healthy Bones

1   Institut national de santé publique du Québec, "From Tiny Tot to Toddler: A Practical Guide for Parents from Pregnancy to Age Two" (2012): 313–530, http://www.inspq.qc.ca/tinytot.

2   Fédération des producteurs de lait du Québec http://www.

lafamilledulait.com/publivores/36-un_verre_de_lait_cest_bien_mais_deux_cest_mieux.

3   "Milk Boy in A Mirror Ad from 1992," made by the National Dairy Board, posted by user "ClassicCommercials4U," December 16, 2008, https://www.youtube.com/watch?v=0G6JymgFusw&feature=youtu.be.

4   Hominidés.com: Les évolutions de l'homme, "Le séquençage du génome du chimpanzé!" September 2005, http://www.hominides.com/html/actualites/actu080905-adn-chimpanze.php.

5   PasseportSanté.net, "L'ostéoporose," http://www.passeportsante.net/fr/Maux/Problemes/Fiche.aspx?doc=osteoporose_pm.

6   A. J. Lanou, S. E. Berkow, and N. D. Barnard, "Calcium, Dairy Products, and Bone Health in Children and Young Adults: A Reevaluation of the Evidence," *Pediatrics* 115, no. 3 (March 2005): 736–43.

7   World Health Organization, *Diet, Nutrition and the Prevention of Chronic Diseases — Report of a Joint WHO/FAO Expert Consultation,* 2003, http://www.fao.org/WAIRDOCS/WHO/AC911F/AC911F00.HTM.

8   Health Canada, "Vitamin D and Calcium: Updated Dietary Reference Intakes," March 22, 2012. http://www.hc-sc.gc.ca/fn-an/nutrition/vitamin/vita-d-eng.php.

9   Dietitians of Canada, "Food Sources of Calcium," May 8, 2014, http://www.dietitians.ca/Your-Health/Nutrition-A-Z/Calcium/Food-Sources-of-Calcium.aspx.

10 T. Colin Campbell and Thomas M. Campbell, *The China Study: The Most Comprehensive Study of Nutrition Ever Conducted and the Startling Implications for Diet, Weight Loss, and Long-Term Health* (Dallas: BenBella Books, 2004).

11 Ibid., 205–6.

12 L. A. Frassetto et al., "Worldwide Incidence of Hip Fracture in Elderly Women: Relation to Consumption of Animal and Vegetable Foods," *Journal of Gerontology: Medical Sciences* 55, no. 10 (October 2000): M585–92.

13 N. M. Maalouf et al., "Hypercalciuria Associated with High Dietary Protein Intake Is Not Due to Acid Load," *Journal of Clinical Endocrinology and Metabolism* 96, no. 12 (December 2011): 3733–40.

14 J. E. Kerstetter, A. M. Kenny, and K. L. Insogna, "Dietary Protein

and Skeletal Health: A Review of Recent Human Research," *Current Opinion in Lipidology* 22, no. 1 (February 2011): 16–20.

15　J. E. Kerstetter et al., "The Impact of Dietary Protein on Calcium Absorption and Kinetic Measures of Bone Turnover in Women," *Journal of Clinical Endocrinology and Metabolism* 90, no. 1 (January 2005): 26–31.

16　Email exchange between the author and Dr. Michael Greger, August 14, 2012.

17　Institute of Medicine of the National Academies, "Dietary Reference Intakes for Calcium and Vitamin D," November 30, 2010, http://iom.nationalacademies.org/reports/2010/dietary-reference-intakes-for-calcium-and-vitamin-d.aspx.

18　Almost all of the United States's milk supply is voluntarily fortified with 100 IU/cup, while in Canada, milk is fortified by law with 35–40 IU/100 mL, as is margarine at ≥530 IU/100 g. National Institutes of Health, "Vitamin D," November 10, 2014, http://ods.od.nih.gov/factsheets/VitaminD-HealthProfessional.

19　D. Feskanich, W. C. Willett, and G. A. Colditz, "Calcium, Vitamin D, Milk Consumption, and Hip Fractures: A Prospective Study among Postmenopausal Women," *American Journal of Clinical Nutrition* 77, no. 2 (February 2003): 504–11.

20　*L'épicerie*, "Le nouveau Guide alimentaire canadien," ICI Radio-Canada, television broadcast on March 7, 2007, http://www.radio-canada.ca/actualite/v2/lepicerie/niveau2_14082.shtml.

21　Pierre Lefrançois, "Vitamine D: des chercheurs suggèrent un apport quotidien de 2000 UI par jour," PasseportSanté.net, June 17, 2009, http://www.passeportsante.net/fr/Actualites/Nouvelles/Fiche.aspx?doc=2009061680_vitamine-d-des-chercheurs-suggerent-un-apport-quotidien-de-2000-ui-par-jour.

22　D. A. Hanley and K. S. Davison, "Vitamin D Insufficiency in North America," *The Journal of Nutrition* 135, no. 2 (February 2005): 332–37.

23　PasseportSanté.net, "Vitamine D," January 2014, http://www.passeportsante.net/fr/Solutions/PlantesSupplements/Fiche.aspx?doc=vitamine_d_ps.

24　T. C. Chen et al., "Factors that Influence the Cutaneous Synthesis and Dietary Sources of Vitamin D," *Archives of Biochemistry and Biophysics* 460, no. 2 (April 15, 2007): 213–17.

25　Stephen Brook, "Vegans Force Nestlé Climbdown," *Guardian*,

September 28, 2005, http://www.theguardian.com/media/2005/sep/28/advertising.

26 PasseportSanté.net, "Le calcium est essentiel . . . Et le lait?" http://www.passeportsante.net/fr/Actualites/Dossiers/ArticleComplementaire.aspx?doc=lait_calcium_do.

27 P. Weber, "Vitamin K and Bone Health," *Nutrition* 17, no. 10 (October 2001): 880–87.

28 PasseportSanté.net, "Lait," http://www.passeportsante.net/fr/Nutrition/EncyclopedieAliments/Fiche.aspx?doc=lait_nu.

29 Lise Bergeron, "Boissons de soya, de riz, d'amandes . . . Que choisir?" Protégezvous.ca, September 2012, http://www.protegez-vous.ca/boissons-vegetales.html.

30 Soya.be, "History of Soybeans," http://www.soya.be/history-of-soybeans.php.

31 Physicians Committee for Responsible Medicine, "The Protein Myth," http://www.pcrm.org/health/diets/vegdiets/how-can-i-get-enough-protein-the-protein-myth.

32 Marie Allard, "Encore plus d'OGM dans nos champs," *La Presse*, July 4, 2011, http://www.lapresse.ca/actualites/201107/03/01-4414689-encore-plus-dogm-dans-noschamps.php.

33 Veronique Dupont, "GMO Corn, Soybeans Dominate US Market," Phys.org, June 4, 2013, http://phys.org/news/2013-06-gmo-corn-soybeans-dominate.html.

34 Élise Desaulniers, *Je mange avec ma tête: Les consequences de nos choix alimentaires* (Montreal: Stanké, 2011), 132–33.

35 N. Guha et al., "Soy Isoflavones and Risk of Cancer Recurrence in a Cohort of Breast Cancer Survivors: The Life After Cancer Epidemiology Study," *Breast Cancer Research and Treatment* 118, no. 2 (November 2009): 395–405.

36 X. O. Shu et al., "Soy Food Intake and Breast Cancer Survival," *JAMA* 302, no. 22 (December 9, 2009): 2437–43.

37 B. J. Caan et al., "Soy Food Consumption and Breast Cancer Prognosis," *Cancer Epidemiology, Biomarkers & Prevention* 20, no. 5 (May 2011): 854–58.

38 Joseph Gonzales, "Should I Stay Away from Soy If I Have Breast Cancer?" NutritionFacts.org, March 4, 2015, http://nutritionfacts.org/rdquestions/should-i-stay-away-from-soy-if-i-have-breast-cancer/.

39 *Fox News*, "Study: Eating Soy May Decrease Sperm Count in Men," October 18, 2007, http://www.foxnews.com/story/2007/10/18/study-eating-soy-may-decrease-sperm-count-in-men.html.

40 Justine Butler, "Ignore the Anti-Soya Scaremongers," *Guardian*, July 1, 2010, http://www.theguardian.com/commentisfree/2010/jul/01/anti-soya-brigade-ignore-scaremongering.

41 J. E. Chavarro et al., "Soy Food and Isoflavone Intake in Relation to Semen Quality Parameters among Men from an Infertility Clinic," *Human Reproduction* 23, no. 11 (November 2008): 2584–90.

42 Virginia Messina, MPH, RD, "Safety of Soyfoods," Vegetarian Nutrition, a dietetic practice group of the Academy of Nutrition and Dietetics, 2012, http://vegetariannutrition.net/docs/Soy-Safety.pdf.

Chapter 3: One Glass of Milk Is Good, but Two Is Better

1 Benjamin Spock, MD, "Good Nutrition for Kids," *Good Medicine* VII, no. 2 (Spring/Summer 1998), http://www3.ul.ie/~sextonb/foodforthought/spock.htm.

2 Heidi Splete, "USDA Panel Skeptical about Milk's Health Claims," *Family Practice News* 31, no. 24 (December 15, 2001): 12.

3 Quoted in Rob Cunningham, *Smoke & Mirrors: The Canadian Tobacco War* (Ottawa, ON, Canada: International Development Research Centre, 1996), 80.

4 See Timothy E. Simalenga and R. Anne Pearson's *Using Cows for Work*, August 2003, http://www.vet.ed.ac.uk/ctvm/Research/DAPR/Training%20Publications/Cows%20%20001/9202_Using_Cows.pdf.

5 Frédéric Forge, "Recombinant Bovine Somatotropin (rbST)," Science and Technology Division, Parliamentary Research Branch, Government of Canada, October 1998, http://publications.gc.ca/collections/Collection-R/LoPBdP/BP/prb981-e.htm.

6 K. Maruyama, T. Oshima, and K. Ohyama, "Exposure to Exogenous Estrogen Through Intake of Commercial Milk Produced from Pregnant Cows," *Pediatrics International* 52, no. 1 (February 2010): 33–38.

7 Ibid.

8 Nicholas Bakalar, "Rise in Rate of Twin Births May Be Tied to Dairy Case," *New York Times*, May 30, 2006, http://www.nytimes.com/2006/05/30/health/30twin.html?_r=0.

9 B. C. Melnik, "Evidence for Acne-Promoting Effects of Milk and

Other Insulinotropic Dairy," *Nestlé Nutrition Workshop Series: Pediatric Program* 67 (2011): 131–45.

10 Joseph Keon, op. cit., 34.

11 C. A. Adebamowo et al., "High School Dietary Dairy Intake and Teenage Acne," *Journal of the American Academy of Dermatology* 52, no. 2 (February 2005): 207–14.

12 C. A. Adebamowo et al., "Milk Consumption and Acne in Adolescent Girls," *Dermatology Online Journal* 12, no. 4 (May 30, 2006): 1.

13 D. Ganmaa et al., "Incidence and Mortality of Testicular and Prostatic Cancers in Relation to World Dietary Practices," *International Journal of Cancer* 98, no. 2 (March 10, 2002): 262–67.

14 D. Ganmaa and A. Sato, "The Possible Role of Female Sex Hormones in Milk from Pregnant Cows in the Development of Breast, Ovarian and Corpus Uteri Cancers," *Medical Hypotheses* 65, no. 6 (2005): 1028–37.

15 D. Ganmaa et al., "Is Milk Responsible for Male Reproductive Disorders?" *Medical Hypotheses* 57, no. 4 (October 2001): 510–14.

16 M. T. Brinkman et al., "Consumption of Animal Products, Their Nutrient Components and Postmenopausal Circulating Steroid Hormone Concentrations," *European Journal of Clinical Nutrition* 64, no. 2 (February 2010): 176–83.

17 Michael Huncharek et al. "Colorectal Cancer Risk and Dietary Intake of Calcium, Vitamin D, and Dairy Products: A Meta-analysis of 26,335 Cases from 60 Observational Studies," *Nutrition and Cancer* 61, no. 1 (2009): 47–69.

18 Joseph Keon, op. cit., 58.

19 Jeanine M. Genkinger et al., "Dairy Products and Ovarian Cancer: A Pooled Analysis of 12 Cohort Studies," *Cancer Epidemiology, Biomarkers & Prevention* 15, no. 2 (February 2006): 364–72.

20 Joseph Keon, op. cit., 65.

21 Ibid., 67.

22 H. A. Sampson, "Update on Food Allergy," *Journal of Allergy and Clinical Immunology* 113, no. 5 (May 2004): 805–19.

23 Association québécoise des allergies alimentaires, "Statistiques," http://allergies-alimentaires.org/fr/statistiques.

24 Joseph Keon, op. cit., 37.

25 Association québécoise des allergies alimentaires, op. cit.

26 Centre d'Information et de Recherche sur les Intolérances et

l'Hygiène Alimentaires, "L'allergie aux protéines du lait de vache et l'intolérance au lactose," http://www.ciriha.org/index.php/allergies-et-intolerances/l-allergie-aux-proteines-du-lait-de-vache-et-l-intolerance-au-lactose.

27 C. S. Williamson, "Nutrition in Pregnancy," *British Nutrition Foundation Nutrition Bulletin* 31, no. 1 (March 2006): 28–59.

28 E. Birch et al., "Breast-Feeding and Optimal Visual Development," *Journal of Pediatric Ophthalmology and Strabismus* 30, no. 1 (January–February 1993): 33–38.

29 M. Makrides et al., "Erythrocyte Docosahexaenoic Acid Correlates with the Visual Response of Healthy, Term Infants," *Pediatric Research* 33, no. 4 pt. 1 (April 1993): 425–27.

30 M. H. Jørgensen et al., "Visual Acuity and Erythrocyte Docosahexaenoic Acid Status in Breast-Fed and Formula-Fed Term Infants During the First Four Months of Life," *Lipids* 31, no. 1 (January 1996): 99–105.

31 S. Lucarelli et al., "Food Allergy and Infantile Autism," *Panminerva Medica* 37, no. 3 (September 1995): 137–41.

32 Joseph Keon, op. cit.

33 D. Ratner, E. Shoshani, and B. Dubnov, "Milk Protein-Free Diet for Nonseasonal Asthma and Migraine in Lactase-Deficient Patients," *Israel Journal of Medical Science* 19, no. 9 (September 1983): 806–9.

34 H. Juntti et al., "Cow's Milk Allergy Is Associated with Recurrent Otitis Media During Childhood," *Acta Oto-Laryngologica* 119, no. 8 (1999): 867–73.

35 T. M. Nsouli et al., "Role of Food Allergy in Serous Otitis Media," *Annals of Allergy* 73, no. 3 (September 1994): 215–19.

36 A. L. Parke and G. R. Hughes, "Rheumatoid Arthritis and Food: A Case Study," *British Medical Journal* 282 no. 6281 (June 20, 1981): 2027–29.

37 Joseph Keon, op. cit., 146.

38 Ibid.

39 K. Dahl-Jørgensen, G. Joner, and K. F. Hanssen, "Relationship Between Cows' Milk Consumption and Incidence of IDDM in Childhood," *Diabetes Care* 14, no. 11 (November 1991): 1081–83.

40 Barbara Kamer et al., "Intestinal Colic in Infants in the First Three Months of Life—Based on Own Observations," *Gastroenterologia Polska* 17, no. 5 (2010): 351–54.

41 K. D. Lust, J. E. Brown, and W. Thomas, "Maternal Intake of

Cruciferous Vegetables and Other Foods and Colic Symptoms in Exclusively Breast-fed Infants," *Journal of the American Dietetic Association* 96, no. 1 (January 1996): 46–48.

42   Dairy Goodness, "Lactose: Simple Tips for Tolerance," http://www.dairygoodness.ca/good-health/dairy-facts-fallacies/lactose-simple-tips-for-tolerance.

43   Health Canada, "Nutrient Value of Some Common Foods," 2008, http://www.hc-sc.gc.ca/fn-an/nutrition/fiche-nutri-data/nutrient_value-valeurs_nutritives-tc-tm-eng.php.

44   U. S. Food and Drug Administration, "Eat for a Healthy Heart," http://www.fda.gov/forconsumers/consumerupdates/ucm199058.htm.

45   S. S. Soedamah-Muthu et al., "Milk and Dairy Consumption and Incidence of Cardiovascular Diseases and All-Cause Mortality: Dose-Response Meta-analysis of Prospective Cohort Studies," *American Journal of Clinical Nutrition* 93, no. 1 (January 2011): 158–71.

46   A. M. Bernstein et al., "Major Dietary Protein Sources and Risk of Coronary Heart Disease in Women," *Circulation* 122 (2010): 876–83.

47   PasseportSanté.net, "Guide alimentaire canadien," http://www.passeportsante.net/fr/Nutrition/Regimes/Fiche.aspx?doc=guide_alimentaire_canadien_regime.

48   Rob Stein, "Study: More Milk Means More Weight Gain," *Washington Post*, June 7, 2005, http://www.washingtonpost.com/wp-dyn/content/article/2005/06/06/AR2005060601348.html.

49   Carolyn W. Gunther, "Dairy Products Do Not Lead to Alterations in Body Weight or Fat Mass in Young Women in a 1-Y Intervention," *American Journal of Clinical Nutrition* 81, no. 4 (April 2005): 751–56.

50   Joseph Keon, op. cit., 81–82.

51   Kim Severson, "Dairy Council to End Ad Campaign that Linked Drinking Milk with Weight Loss," *New York Times*, May 11, 2007, http://www.nytimes.com/2007/05/11/us/11milk.html.

52   C. S. Berkey et al., "Milk, Dairy Fat, Dietary Calcium, and Weight Gain: A Longitudinal Study of Adolescents," *Archives of Pediatrics and Adolescent Medicine* 159, no. 6 (June 2005): 543–50.

53   University of Ottawa, "Sudden Infant Death Syndrome in Canada," January 13, 2015, http://www.med.uottawa.ca/sim/data/SIDS_e.htm.

54 Z. Sun et al., "Relation of Beta-Casomorphin to Apnea in Sudden Infant Death Syndrome," *Peptides* 24, no. 6 (June 2003): 937–43.

55 J. Wasilewska et al., "Cow's-Milk-Induced Infant Apnoea with Increased Serum Content of Bovine β-Casomorphin-5," *Journal of Pediatric Gastroenterology and Nutrition* 52, no. 6 (June 2011): 772–75.

56 W. E. Parish et al., "Hypersensitivity to Milk and Sudden Death in Infancy," *The Lancet* 276, no. 7160 (November 19, 1960): 1106–10.

57 M. Park et al., "Consumption of Milk and Calcium in Midlife and the Future Risk of Parkinson Disease," *Neurology* 64, no. 6 (March 22, 2005): 1047–51.

58 H. Chen et al., "Consumption of Dairy Products and Risk of Parkinson's Disease," *American Journal of Epidemiology* 165, no. 9 (May 1, 2007): 998–1006.

59 Joseph Keon, op. cit., 69.

60 Keith Woodford, *Devil in the Milk: Illness, Health, and the Politics of A1 and A2 Milk* (White River Junction, VT: Chelsea Green Publishing, 2009).

61 At the Université Laval, for example, medical students have no mandatory nutrition course during their general training. The only course offered is optional. Université Laval, "Doctor of Medicine (MD)," http://www2.ulaval.ca/les-etudes/programmes/repertoire/details/doctorat-en-medecine-md.html.

62 New York Times Syndicate, "Go Heavy on the Veggies to Prevent Cancer," *Aetna*, July 21, 1999, cited by Keon, op. cit., 240, note 7.

63 J. S. Goodwin and J. M. Goodwin, "The Tomato Effect: Rejection of Highly Efficacious Therapies," *JAMA* 251, no. 18 (May 11, 1984): 2387–90.

64 Quoted by Jacqueline Lagacé, op. cit., 232.

Chapter 4: We Can Trust the Experts

1 Dairy Nutrition, "Scientific Evidence," http://www.dairynutrition.ca/scientific-evidence.

2 National Dairy Council, "Misperceptions Regarding Dairy Foods: A Review of the Evidence," *Dairy Council Digest* 81, no. 1 (January–February 2010), http://www.nationaldairycouncil.org/SiteCollectionDocuments/child_nutrition/health_kit/dcd811.pdf.

3   Harvard School of Public Health, "Food Pyramids and Plates: What Should You Really Eat?" http://www.hsph.harvard.edu/nutritionsource/pyramid-full-story/.

4   Dairy Nutrition, "Milk Products: An Important Tool for Weight Management," http://www.dairynutrition.ca/scientific-evidence/experts-summaries/milk-products-an-important-tool-for-weight-management.

5   Peter Boyle et al., eds. *Tobacco: Science, Policy, and Public Health*, Second Edition (New York: Oxford University Press, 2010), 62.

6   Justin E. Bekelman, Yan Li, and Cary P. Gross, "Scope and Impact of Financial Conflicts of Interest in Biomedical Research: A Systematic Review," *JAMA* 289, no. 4 (2003): 454–65.

7   Cat Warren, "Big Food, Big Agra, and the Research University," *Academe*, November–December 2010, http://www.aaup.org/aaup/pubsres/academe/2010/nd/feat/nest.htm.

8   For more information on the dairy industry's contributions to health research, visit http://www.dairynutrition.ca/research-funding.

9   Marion Nestle, *Food Politics: How the Food Industry Influences Nutrition and Health* (Oakland: University of California Press, 2002), xv.

10   L. I. Lesser et al., "Relationship Between Funding Source and Conclusion among Nutrition-Related Scientific Articles," *PLOS Medicine* 4, no. 1 (January 9, 2007): e5.

11   M. B. Katan, "Does Industry Sponsorship Undermine the Integrity of Nutrition Research?" *PLOS Medicine* 4, no. 1 (January 9, 2007): e6.

12   "Danone règle une poursuite concernant le yogourt Activia," *Argent*, September 24, 2012, http://argent.canoe.ca/lca/affaires/canada/archives/2012/09/Danone-poursuite-yogourt-Activia.html.

13   Annie Morin, "Yogourt santé au Canada, mais pas en Europe," *Le Soleil*, April 20, 2010, http://www.lapresse.ca/le-soleil/affaires/agro-alimentaire/201004/19/01-4272157-yogourt-sante-au-canada-mais-pas-en-europe.php.

14   Felicity Lawrence, "Are Probiotics Really That Good for Your Health?" *Guardian*, July 24, 2009, http://www.theguardian.com/theguardian/2009/jul/25/probiotic-health-benefits.

15 Dairy Farmers of Canada, "Guidelines for Research Funding," http://www.dairynutrition.ca/content/download/256/2128/version/147/file/GUIDELINES-FOR-GRANT-APPLICATION-2015.pdf.

16 Cat Warren, op. cit.

Chapter 5: Schoolchildren Need Milk

1 Valéry Colas, "La crise, les écoliers et l'accès au lait," *Cap-aux-Diamants: la revue d'histoire du Québec* 71 (automne 2002): 35.

2 Ibid.

3 Annie Morin, "Plaidoyer pour le retour du berlingot de lait," *Le Soleil*, April 17, 2009, http://www.lapresse.ca/le-soleil/affaires/agro-alimentaire/200904/16/01-847341-plaidoyer-pour-le-retour-du-berlingot-de-lait.php.

4 Ibid.

5 La famille du Lait, "Tournée dans les écoles—Grand Défi Pierre Lavoie," http://lafamilledulait.com/evenements/tournee-dans-les-ecoles-grand-defi-pierre-lavoie.

6 Center for Science in the Public Interest, "The 1% Or Less School Kit," https://www.cspinet.org/nutrition/schoolkit.html.

7 Canadian Digestive Health Foundation, "Statistics," http://www.cdhf.ca/en/statistics.

8 Michele Simon, *Whitewashed: How Industry and Government Promote Dairy Junk Foods*, Eat Drink Politics, June 2014, http://www.eatdrinkpolitics.com/wp-content/uploads/SimonWhitewashedDairyReport.pdf.

9 Ibid.

10 Hélène Baribeau, "Trop de sucre: où est la limite?" PasseportSanté.net, http://www.passeportsante.net/fr/actualites/dossiers/articlecomplementaire.aspx?doc=sucre_limite_consommation_do.

11 Marie Allard, "Faut-il interdire le lait au chocolat à l'école," *La Presse*, May 13, 2011, http://www.lapresse.ca/vivre/sante/nutrition/201105/13/01-4399004-faut-il-interdire-le-lait-auchocolat-a-lecole.php.

12 Hélène Baribeau, op. cit.

13 The Food Revolution Team, "A Recipe for Change: Flavored Milk HQ," Jamie Oliver Food Foundation USA, October 19, 2011, http://www.jamieoliverfoodfoundation.org/usa/news-content/a-recipe-for-change-flavored-milk-1.

14 Protégez-vous, "Yogourts à boire ou en tube: 4 produits évalués," http://www.protegez-vous.ca/sante-et-alimentation/yogourts-aux-fraises/yogourts-a-boire-ou-en-tube-4-produits-evalues. html. (Subscription required.)

15 Gouvernement du Québec, *Plan d'action gouvernemental de promotion des saines habitudes de vie et de prévention des problèmes reliés au poids 2006–2012 — Investir pour l'avenir*, October 23, 2006, http://msssa4.msss.gouv.qc.ca/fr/document/publication.

16 Éric Giroux, "Eduquer et vendre: la Santé par le Lait Inc.," *Cap-aux-Diamants: la revue d'histoire du Québec* 71 (automne 2002): 38.

17 Ibid., 44.

18 Ibid., 45.

19 Ibid., 45.

20 Nicole Dubé, "Avec le temps, le lait apported son lot de souvenirs: les secret d'un marketing efficace," *Cap-aux-Diamants: la revue d'histoire du Québec* 71 (automne 2002): 49.

21 Ibid., 50.

22 Ibid., 51.

23 La famille du Lait, "La campagne blanche," 2001, http://lafamilledulait.com/publivores/la-campagne-blanche.

Chapter 6: If Cows Were Unhappy, They Wouldn't Produce Milk

1 Étienne Gosselin, "Un Québec entravé dans un Canada libre," *Cooperateur*, February 2012, http://www.lacoop.coop/cooperateur/articles/2012/02/p36.asp.

2 USDA, "Dairy 2007: Facility Characteristics and Cow Comfort on U.S. Dairy Operations," http://www.aphis.usda.gov/animal_health/nahms/dairy/downloads/dairy07/Dairy07_ir_Facilities.pdf.

3 Étienne Gosselin, op. cit.

4 Marie Allard, "Les vaches du Québec sont confinées à l'étable," *La Presse*, August 31, 2012, http://www.lapresse.ca/actualites/quebec-canada/national/201208/31/01-4569963-les-vaches-du-quebec-sont-confinees-a-letable.php.

5 University of British Columbia Dairy Education and Research Center, "What Cows Prefer: Pasture and Access to the Barn," *Research Reports* 10, no. 3 (May 2010), http://www.farmwest.com/images/clientpdfs/ResearchVol10No3.pdf.

6   Élise Desaulniers, op. cit., 39.

7   Alexis C. Madrigal, "The Perfect Milk Machine: How Big Data Transformed the Dairy Industry," *The Atlantic*, May 1, 2012, http://www.theatlantic.com/technology/archive/2012/05/the-perfect-milk-machine-how-big-data-transformed-the-dairy-industry/256423/.

8   John Webster, *Understanding the Dairy Cow*, Second Edition (Oxford, UK: Blackwell Scientific Publications, 1993). Quoted in Nigel B. Cook, "Time Budgets for Dairy Cows: How Does Cow Comfort Influence Health, Reproduction and Productivity?" (University of Wisconsin, Madison School of Veterinary Medicine), http://www.vetmed.wisc.edu/dms/fapm/publicats/proceeds/timebudgetsanddairycowsomaha.pdf.

9   Email exchange between the author and Dr. Olivier Berreville, July 2012.

10 I. R. Dohoo et al., "A Meta-analysis Review of the Effects of Recombinant Bovine Somatotropin," *Canadian Journal of Veterinary Research* 67, no. 4 (October 2003): 252–64.

11 Daniel Roussel, "Vos vaches se plaignent-elles d'acidose?" *Le producteur de lait québécois* (April 2008): 26, https://www.yumpu.com/fr/document/view/30111629/vos-vaches-se-plaignent-elles-dacidose.

12 Martin Ménard, "Le bien-être animal et les vaches laitières," *L'Utiliterre*, May 26, 2011, http://www.laterre.ca/actualites/elevages/le-bien-etre-animal-et-les-vaches-laitieres.php.

13 Centre d'insémination artificielle du Québec (CIAQ), "Who Is Starbuck?" http://www.ciaq.com/ciaq/history/the-legend-of-starbuck/who-is-starbuck.html.

14 Traci Hobson, "Factory Farming in America, Part 5: The Life of a Dairy Cow," Ian Somerhalder Foundation, http://www.isfoundation.com/campaign/factory-farming-america-part-5-life-dairy-cow.

15 Megan Cross, "Mother Cow Proves Animals Love, Think & Act," *Global Animal*, April 13, 2012, http://www.globalanimal.org/2012/04/13/cow-proves-animals-love-think-andact/71867.

16 Ibid.

17 Pat Donworth, "The Secret Life of Moody Cows," Golden Age of Gaia, August 14, 2011, http://goldenageofgaia.com/2011/08/the-secret-life-of-moody-cows.

18   Rosamund Young, *The Secret Life of Cows* (Preston, UK: Good Life Press, 2003).

19   Julianna Kettlewell, "Farm Animals 'Need Emotional TLC,'" *BBC News*, March 18, 2005, http://news.bbc.co.uk/2/hi/science/nature/4360947.stm.

20   "The Great Escape," RTÉ News, June 15, 2011, http://www.rte.ie/news/2011/0615/cow.html.

21   Pierre-Paul Noreau, "Abattoir Levinoff-Colbex: fermer le robinet," *Le Soleil*, May 30, 2012, http://www.lapresse.ca/le-soleil/opinions/editoriaux/201205/29/01-4529813-abattoir-levinoff-colbex-fermer-le-robinet.php.

22   Annie Morin, "Fermeture de Levinoff-Colbex: les bêtes devront être abattues en Ontario," *Le Soleil*, May 30, 2012, http://www.lapresse.ca/le-soleil/affaires/agro-alimentaire/201205/29/01-4529860-fermeture-de-levinoff-colbex-les-betes-devront-etre-abattues-en-ontario.php.

23   Timothy Pachirat, *Every Twelve Seconds: Industrialized Slaughter and the Politics of Sight* (New Haven, CT: Yale University Press, 2011).

24   Gary L. Francione, *Animals as Persons: Essays on the Abolition of Animal Exploitation* (New York: Columbia University Press, 2008), 108.

25   Melanie Joy, *Why We Love Dogs, Eat Pigs, and Wear Cows: An Introduction to Carnism* (San Francisco: Conari Press, 2009).

26   Vegetarian Resource Group, "Position of the American Dietetic Association and Dieticians of Canada: Vegetarian Diets," *ADA Reports* 103, no. 6 (June 2003): 748–65, http://www.vrg.org/nutrition/2003_ADA_position_paper.pdf.

27   Winston J. Craig and Ann Reed Mangels, "Position of the American Dietetic Association: Vegetarian Diets," *Journal of the American Dietetic Association* 109, no. 7 (July 2009): 1266–82, http://www.vrg.org/nutrition/2009_ADA_position_paper.pdf.

28   Paul Slovic, "'If I Look at the Mass I Will Never Act': Psychic Numbing and Genocide," *Judgment and Decision Making* 2, no. 2 (April 2007): 79–95, http://journal.sjdm.org/jdm7303a.pdf.

29   Author interview with Dr. Martin Gibert, August 2012.

30   See Brock Bastian et al., "Don't Mind Meat? The Denial of Mind to Animals Used for Human Consumption," *Personality and Social Psychology Bulletin* 38, no. 2 (February 2012): 247–56.

31 Sue Donaldson and Will Kymlicka, *Zoopolis: A Political Theory of Animal Rights* (New York: Oxford University Press, 2011).

Chapter 7: Animal Abuse Is Illegal

1   Jocelyne Richer, "Le PQ craint que la viande halal devienne la règle," *La Presse*, March 23, 2012, http://www.lapresse.ca/actualites/quebec-canada/politique-quebecoise/201203/23/01-4508701-le-pq-craint-que-la-viande-halal-devienne-laregle.php.

2   Humane Society International, "HSI Presse le Gouvernement d'Agir—Le Québec Classé Pire Province pour les Animaux," May 19, 2011, http://www.hsi.org/french/news/press_releases/2011/05/Quebec_classe_pire_province_pour_les_animaux_051911.html.

3   Publications du Québec, *Animal Health Protection Act*, chapter P-42, http://www2.publicationsduquebec.gouv.qc.ca/dynamicSearch/telecharge.php?type=2&file=/P_42/P42_A.html.

4   Email exchange between the author and Sophie Gaillard, July 12–13, 2012.

5   World Animal Protection, *What's on Your Plate?: The Hidden Costs of Industrial Animal Agriculture in Canada*, 2012, http://issuu.com/wspacanada/docs/wspa_whatsonyourplate_fullreport.

6   Email exchange between the author and Sophie Gaillard, June 18, 2015.

7   National Farm Animal Care Council, *Code of Practice for the Care and Handling of Dairy Cattle*, 2009, http://www.dairyfarmers.ca/content/download/181/804/version/2/file/Dairy_Code_ENG_March09.pdf.

8   Email exchange between the author and Sophie Gaillard, April 25, 2012.

9   CIAQ, "Saisir les opportunités pour faire un bon 'coût'!" October 27, 2011, http://www.ciaq.com/actualites/nouvelles/2011/saisir-les-opportunites-pour-faire-un-bon-cout.html.

10 Michel Lemire, "Confortablement lait!" 35e Symposium sur les Bovins laitiers, October 27, 2011, http://www.agrireseau.qc.ca/bovinslaitiers/documents/Lemire.pdf.

Chapter 8: Cheese Is Green

1   Marc Allard, "Jour 7: La bière et les mains vides," *Le Soleil*,

December 1, 2008, http://www.lapresse.ca/le-soleil/dossiers/changer-sa-vie/200812/01/01-806032-jour-7-la-biere-et-les-mains-vides.php.

2   Marc Allard, "Jour 28: Du lait bio, et après? (2e partie)," *Le Soleil*, December 22, 2008, http://www.lapresse.ca/le-soleil/dossiers/changer-sa-vie/200812/22/01-812465-jour-28-du-lait-bio-et-apres-2e-partie.php.

3   Organic Agriculture Centre of Canada, "Raising Calves on Organic Dairy Farms," July 2009, http://www.organicagcentre.ca/DOCs/AnimalWelfare/AWTF/Dairy_calves.pdf.

4   Jean Durocher, Francois Labelle, and Guillaume Bergeron, "Santé du pis et production laitière biologique—La clé de la stratégie: La prevention!" Valacta, September 2010, http://www.agrireseau.qc.ca/agriculturebiologique/documents/valacta_prevention_key_f[1].pdf.

5   Sonia Gosselin, "Démystifier le bio!" Valacta, http://www.agrireseau.qc.ca/agriculturebiologique/documents/D%C3%A9mystifier%20le%20bio12.15.11__.pdf.

6   Geneviève Blain, *Recommandation de mise en marché pour les bovins de réforme biologiques*, Syndicat des producteurs de viande biologique du Québec, http://www.agrireseau.qc.ca/agriculturebiologique/documents/Rapport%20final%2007-BIO-02.pdf.

7   See http://www.meatlessmonday.com/.

8   Food and Agriculture Organization of the United Nations, *Livestock's Long Shadow: Environmental Issues and Options*, 2009, http://www.fao.org/docrep/010/a0701e/a0701e00.htm.

9   Kari Hamerschlag, *Meat Eater's Guide to Climate Change and Health*, Environmental Working Group, July 2011, http://static.ewg.org/reports/2011/meateaters/pdf/report_ewg_meat_eaters_guide_to_health_and_climate_2011.pdf.

10   Environmental Working Group, "Climate and Environmental Impacts," http://www.ewg.org/meateatersguide/a-meat-eaters-guide-to-climate-change-health-what-you-eat-matters/climate-and-environmental-impacts/.

11   Time for Change, "What Is A Carbon Footprint—Definition," http://timeforchange.org/what-is-a-carbon-footprint-definition.

12   Nina Shen Rastogi, "Different Cheeses Have Varying Environmental Impacts; Sheep Cheese Is Harshest," *Washington*

Post, December 15, 2009, http://www.washingtonpost.com/wp-dyn/content/article/2009/12/14/AR2009121402880.html.

13 Lisa Hymas, "Is Your Cheese Killing the Planet?" *Mother Jones*, August 10, 2011, http://www.motherjones.com/bluemarble/2011/08/your-cheese-killing-planet.

14 Annika Smedman et al., "Nutrient Density of Beverages in Relation to Climate Impact," *Food & Nutrition Research* 54 (2010): 5170.

15 Food and Agriculture Organization of the United Nations, Animal Production and Health Division, *Greenhouse Gas Emissions from the Dairy Sector: A Life Cycle Assessment*, 2010, http://www.fao.org/docrep/012/k7930e/k7930e00.pdf.

16 Environment Canada, *National Inventory Report, Greenhouse Gas Sources and Sinks in Canada 1990–2010*, http://ec.gc.ca/publications/A91164E0-7CEB-4D61-841C-BEA8BAA223F9/Executive-Summary-2012_WEB-v3.pdf.

17 USDA Economic Research Service, "Irrigation and Water Use—Background, " June 7, 2013, http://www.ers.usda.gov/topics/farm-practices-management/irrigation-water-use/background.aspx.

18 Nathan Runkle, "Cheeseburgers, Climate Change and the California Drought," *Huffington Post*, May 12, 2015, http://www.huffingtonpost.com/nathan-runkle/cheeseburgers-climate-cha_b_7266354.html.

19 A. Ertug Ercin, Maite M. Aldaya, and Arjen Y. Hoekstra, "The Water Footprint of Soy Milk and Soy Burger and Equivalent Animal Products," *Ecological Indicators* 18 (2012): 392–402.

20 Marc Allard, "Jour 4: La rareté rend gai," *Le Soleil*, November 28, 2008, http://www.lapresse.ca/le-soleil/dossiers/changer-sa-vie/200811/28/01-805236-jour-4-la-rarete-rend-gai.php.

21 Christopher L. Weber and H. Scott Matthews, "Food-Miles and the Relative Climate Impacts of Food Choices in the United States," *Environmental Science and Technology* 4, no. 10 (2008): 3508–13.

Chapter 9: It's an Industry Just Like Any Other

1 Jean-Marc Léger, "Le baromètre des professions," *Le Journal de Montréal*, September, 29, 2010.

2 Dairy Farmers of Canada, "About Us," http://www.dairyfarmers.ca/who-we-are/about-us.

3   William B. P. Robson and Colin Busby, "Freeing up Food: The Ongoing Cost, and Potential Reform, of Supply Management," *C.D. Howe Institute Backgrounder* 128 (April 2010), https://www.cdhowe.org/sites/default/files/attachments/research_papers/mixed//backgrounder_128.pdf.

4   Groupe Ageco, "Prix du quota de lait par provice, Canada, 2004/2005 a 2010/2011," http://www.groupeageco.ca/fr/pdf/stat/PQ4.pdf.

5   GO5, "WTO and Agriculture—Supply Management," http://www.go5quebec.ca/en/gestion.php.

6   Mark Milke, "Canada's Food Cartels versus Consumers," *Fraser Forum* (May/June 2012): 31–33, http://www.fraserinstitute.org/uploadedFiles/fraser-ca/Content/research-news/research/articles/canadas-food-cartels-versus-consumers.pdf.

7   Canadian Dairy Information Centre, "Number of Farms, Dairy Cows and Heifers," http://www.dairyinfo.gc.ca/index_e.php?s1=dff-fcil&s2=farm-ferme&s3=nb.

8   Eco Ressources Consultants for Dairy Farmers of Canada, *The Economic Impact of the Dairy Industry in Canada*, March 2011, http://www.dairyfarmers.ca/content/download/1088/8440/version/5/file/EcoRessourcesDFC2011-Economic-Impact-Canada.pdf.

9   "Les 500 plus grandes entreprises du Québec 2009," *Les Affaires*, July 1, 2009, http://www.lesaffaires.com/archives/generale/les-500-plus-grandes-entreprises-du-qubec-2009/503053.

10   "Hausse des prix du lait," ICI Radio-Canada, February 1, 2011, http://www.radio-canada.ca/nouvelles/Economie/2011/01/31/011-prix-hausse-lait.shtml.

11   Isabelle Lessard, "Le prix du lait irrite," *Agricom* 29, no. 7 (November 16, 2011), http://journalagricom.ca/le-prix-du-lait-irrite/.

12   Sharon Singleton, "Les restaurateurs dénoncent le prix élevé du lait," *TVA Argent*, October 12, 2011, http://argent.canoe.ca/lca/affaires/canada/archives/2011/10/20111012-180422.html.

13   Gaétane Gôté and Félicien Hitayezu, *Dépenses alimentaires des Québécois: dans le commerce de détail en 2013*, Ministère de l'Agriculture, des Pêcheries et de l'Alimentation du Québec, http://www.mapaq.gouv.qc.ca/fr/Publications/DepensesalimentairesACNielsen.pdf.

14   Ibid.

15 Dairy Management Inc., "DMI and the Dairy Checkoff," http://www.dairy.org/about-dmi.

16 Maine Dairy Promotion Board / Maine Dairy and Nutrition Council, "For Farmers," http://drinkmainemilk.org/for-farmers.

17 Michael Moss, "While Warning About Fat, U.S. Pushes Cheese Sales," *New York Times*, November 6, 2010, http://www.nytimes.com/2010/11/07/us/07fat.html.

18 Ibid.

19 Food excluding restaurants, groceries, and alcohol.

20 A. C. Nielsen, *Dépenses de l'industrie laitière*, 2011.

Chapter 10: I Could Never Live Without Cheese

1 Paul Rozin, "Human Food Intake and Choice: Biological, Psychological and Cultural Perspectives," in H. Anderson, J. Blundell, and M. Chiva (eds), *Food Selection: From Genes to Culture* (Paris: Danone Institute, 2002), 7–24.

2 Gordon M. Shepherd, *Neurogastronomy: How the Brain Creates Flavor and Why It Matters* (New York: Columbia University Press, 2012).

3 Ibid., 166.

4 E. Sienkiewicz-Szłapka et al., "Contents of Agonistic and Antagonistic Opioid Peptides in Different Cheese Varieties," *International Dairy Journal* 19, no. 4 (April 2009): 258–63.

5 E. Hazum et al., "Morphine in Cow and Human Milk: Could Dietary Morphine Constitute a Ligand for Specific Morphine (mu) Receptors?" *Science* 213, no. 4511 (August 28, 1981): 1010–12.

6 Neal D. Barnard, *Breaking the Food Seduction: The Hidden Reasons Behind Food Cravings And 7 Steps to End Them Naturally* (New York: St. Martin's Press, 2003).

7 European Food Safety Authority, "Review of the Potential Health Impact of β-Casomorphins and Related Peptides," *EFSA Scientific Report* 231 (January 29, 2009): 1–107.

8 Neal D. Barnard, op. cit.

9 Email exchange between the author and Renan Larue, July 2012. Renan Larue is also the author of *Le végétarisme et ses ennemis* (*Vegetarianism and Its Enemies*) (Paris, FR: PUF, 2015).

10 The Vegan Society, "Definition of Veganism," http://www.

vegansociety.com/try-vegan/definition-veganism.

11   Neal D. Barnard, op. cit., 69.

12   La Presse Canadienne Montreal, "Le fromage, produit local préféré des Québécois," *Le Soleil*, February 28, 2010, http://www.lapresse.ca/le-soleil/affaires/agro-alimentaire/201002/28/01-4256112-le-fromage-produit-local-prefere-des-quebecois.php.

13   Canadian Dairy Information Centre, "Consumption of Dairy Products," http://www.dairyinfo.gc.ca/index_e.php?s1=dff-fcil&s2=cons&s3=conscdn.

14   Inspired by Neal Barnard, op. cit.

About the Author

Élise Desaulniers is an independent scholar and animal rights activist who published her first book on food ethics, *Je mange avec ma tête* ("I Eat With My Head"), in 2011. She co-authored two articles in the *Encyclopedia of Food and Agricultural Ethics* (Springer 2014) and won the Quebec Grand Prize for independent journalism (opinion), for a piece on feminism and anti-speciesism in 2015. A frequent lecturer and presenter at colleges and universities, she lives in Montreal. To reach the author and stay informed of her latest news: elise.desaulniers@gmail.com; twitter.com/ edesaulniers

About the Publisher

LANTERN BOOKS was founded in 1999 on the principle of living with a greater depth and commitment to the preservation of the natural world. In addition to publishing books on animal advocacy, vegetarianism, religion, and environmentalism, Lantern is dedicated to printing books in the United States on recycled paper and saving resources in day-to-day operations. Lantern is honored to be a recipient of the highest standard in environmentally responsible publishing from the Green Press Initiative.

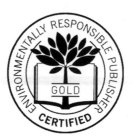

www.lanternbooks.com